Killing Yourself with Your Fork?!

Discover 40 Tips in 40 days to Achieve Maximum Health and Vitality Now!

Francois C. Maloney, MBA, CPCC

iUniverse, Inc.
New York   Bloomington

Killing Yourself with Your Fork?
40 Tips in 40 days to Achieve Maximum Health and Vitality!

iUniverse books may be ordered through booksellers or by contacting:

iUniverse
1663 Liberty Drive
Bloomington, IN 47403
www.iuniverse.com
1-800-Authors (1-800-288-4677)

ISBN: 978-1-4401-3804-1 (sc)
ISBN: 978-1-4401-3806-5 (hc)
ISBN:978-1-4401-3805-8 (ebook)

Printed in the United States of America

iUniverse rev. date: 8/26/2009

Dedication

To my mom who has always believed and supported me in my ability to do anything I set my mind to.

To my late and beloved angel Aida who just passed away, July 12th, 2009. I know you watch over and guide me from beyond. I will always love you and keep you close to my heart, babasaurus!

To my coach Ilan who pushed me and my coaching clients who allowed me to help and learn from. I couldn't have persevered to create this work without all of you. Thank you!

To all the motivational speakers and spiritual leaders who have forged a path and helped me believe in myself enough to write this book, I thank you.

To living a life of joy, freedom and boundless health! You are so worth it!

Contents

1.0 *__Disclosure__*

Neither the content nor the intent of this work may or should be construed as the giving or suggesting of medical advice nor the recommendation of medical treatment of any kind. The information is intended for educational use only and contains the author's opinions and experiences. Its proper purpose is to support informed discussions between patient and health practitioner, to support the concept of genuine cooperation in the patient doctor relationship. It is also to help the patient understand some of the critical concepts behind diet or fitness suggestions and the treatment he or she receives from the doctor. Finally, it is to inform of useful alternative information and to help the reader to identify those health practitioners who keep up with advances in the ever-changing field of health.

1.1 *__Introduction__*

Do you wake up in the morning brimming with energy, literally flying out of bed ready to tackle anything the day throws at you? Or, like most people, do you slam the snooze button continuously in the vain hope of getting some energy to drag yourself up and through the day? I was the second example 2 years ago but I gradually made some dramatic changes and I can now assure you I quite literally jump out of bed every day. Just because you are no longer in your early 20's doesn't mean you need to live a life low in energy and vitality. Forty is the new 30! We hear this all the time. Is it true? If so why do so many people run to pills, injections, facelifts and tummy tucks to relive their 20's? (without the energy and innocence!). Because they don't feel or look good because of their health and diets! If you are still in your 20's, you may be one of the many young people these days who have never felt what full energy feels like or what being healthy is like. Having taken on their parents' bad lifestyle habits, obesity is now a problem in children, perhaps an even greater shame. Many of these young people literally never get a chance to feel or be healthy because they don't know how or why it's important.

" We are not limited by age, we are liberated by it."
Ralph Waldo Emerson

This work is about taking your life, energy and vitality literally in your hands! *This book is a really great start to treating yourself better than you ever have (and do it in a fun and easy way).* This summary of my positive health improvement experiences aims to offer you a compendium of my distillation of many sources to bring to you the critical few things/actions/thoughts you *can and must do/have* to get the results you want in terms of vibrant youthful, health and energy. I've included some relevant quotes where they make sense.

Everything (almost!) you know about energy, food, health and diet is wrong! And, it's not your fault! Through an endless amount of advertising, misinformation, greed and pure manipulation *we are killing ourselves with our forks.* Killing is not a word I use lightly; most of the foods we consume are over- processed, irradiated, dead and quite frankly poisonous. We haven't been taught or given the truth. We eat too much dead, dry food. Over 65% of North Americans are overweight. The top 3 killers are modern diseases and self created: Cancer, Heart Disease/Stroke, and Diabetes. *Not* virulent environmental pathogens (agents) as in past generations (typhoid, influenza, syphilis, etc.). This is the scary side of things. The problem is we are afraid of getting sick (we've been socialized to fear disease by the world. If we take care of our bodies there is very little, actually, nothing, and I mean *nothing* to worry about. *The human body is the most perfect creation* provided the right materials it can withstand incredible conditions and still thrive. The fact that we live on average 80 years *even* with all the horrible things we (modern man) do to it is testament to its durability. If most people treated their cars as they do their bodies, their car would die within months, the human body forges on, never giving up on trying to keep you alive. Once you realize that there are two types of foods, you can choose what you want. One type destroys (clogs) your body, the other type builds (cleans) your body. Most critically, My hope for you is that after reading the book *you will once and for all, stop worrying about your health because you feel incredible always.* Worry, guilt and fear are some of the most destructive emotions you can create/experience (we react to events in our own way, we choose our reaction(s)). So a life of full health, energy and vibrancy/vitality definitely includes a psychological aspect.

"All truth goes through 3 steps: 1st it is ridiculed. 2nd it is violently opposed. Finally it is accepted as self-evident."

A. Schopenhaur

I am not a medical doctor. This is precisely why you should pay attention, I am a regular person, just like you, who has discovered extraordinary results through my own trial and error! My formal education is in business. I have a Bachelor's Degree in Marketing, an MBA in Strategy and have helped hundreds of people in my role as a life design and wellness coach. The fact I have no affiliations or connections with either the fitness, the medical or food industries guarantees I am not connected or complicit financially, ideologically or professionally. This independence allows me a freedom of speech, opinion and experience most professionals in the aforementioned industries could never hope to possess. *People in those industries can not freely or safely disclose without alienating their own peers and communities!* The fact I am relating my own experiences and techniques allows me full liberty. Another great proof of my independence is that this book was self-published allowing me full editorial control of its content.

I have experienced in my body everything I am suggesting to you. I attended an Anthony Robbins "Unleash The Power Within" Seminar[1] last year and learned leading edge information on health. At that time I considered I was very well informed and quite fit, yet I learned so much. I undertook to implement many of the concepts which I found worked brilliantly. My results were incredibly rapid, compelling and dramatic. I discovered that by using my body as the guinea pig, *I became an expert on my health!*

My hope in this work is to have you become the Expert on Your Own health! Who else is as intimately aware of your health? I simply got tired of people asking me some version of "what do you do to look so young and/or have so much energy and/or stay slim?" I realized I was really an expert on my own body and maybe others could learn to do the same. I decided to attempt to write a book based on my experiences, which you now hold in your hands. Thank you for being willing to try something different, you won't be disappointed. I give you my word I've put so much into this and am proud of this book. This (the fact I'm not involved in the health industry) to me is my greatest advantage, I am not caught up in the system of health care on any level, nor is anyone in my family. *I do not own any medical company or natural product stocks nor am I involved in any agreements with any such company.* I am impartial (as relatively as I can imagine) in terms of what I want for you, *massive health now!* I want you to *immediately stop* being afraid of *disease.* What *you should fear* is the manipulation created by the massive "health" and food businesses, both wield immense power. But we also give away our power of information and choice. I want you to make your own choices. I *don't* want you to do anything you don't want to. I want you to try my suggestions yourself for 40 days and feel the difference in your energy, body and decrease or eliminate the ailments you have. With my simple tips you will enjoy eating again and can relax your worry around the amount of food you eat. You will eat more (real food though) without injuring your body as many fad diets do. The rollercoaster of dieting is a crime and you are smarter than that.

"I've been on a diet for 2 weeks and all I've lost is 2 weeks!"
Totie Fields

I aim to teach you to use a much more common sense approach to listening to and treating your body in a way that gives you maximum energy, strength, remove many conditions generally associated with "aging". The key thing I will use is *common sense* something surprisingly few people use it when it comes to how they treat their bodies. I have had the benefit of doing a fair amount of research on the supporting scientific data on what I have lived. I have aimed to simplify my findings for you in a usable format so you can understand it and chose food and exercise intelligently.

I will debunk some myths that frankly you have been advertised and brainwashed for so long it will take an open mind on your part. *Again, use your common sense, if it makes sense use the information I provide.* If not, don't use it. You are the only one in charge of your health, don't give that power away to the media or even friends and family, and look at different options. I have used the principles outlined in this work as a 40 year old man over the last 2 years and have been amazed at how I feel, look and think. I went from a weight of 195 lbs in 2002 to 169 lbs today with the energy, body and sex drive (healthy, great and lots of sex alone is worth the change!) of a typical younger adult. You will feel the impact of these changes *immediately*. After 40 days you will never want to go back! I work out less than I used to, have more energy and get better results due to the (simple to apply) principles you are about to learn! If you follow the crowds around health, you'll get the crowd's results (premature aging, disease, low vitality and worry).

Enough about all that! Let's get to work breaking forward into massive, consistent energy and vibrant health *at any age*. Once you follow core (and easy to follow) principles that create health, energy and a level of newfound optimism around your body. You can now say goodbye to fear forever!

Forget the idea that aging is equal to decreased health, *it's false!* Jack Lalanne (of late night infomercial fame) once did 1033 pushups in 23 minutes at 43. He still works out 90 minutes a day with weights and swims for 30 minutes at 94 years of age.[2]

I have heard of a 70 year old man who bench presses over 400 pounds! *New research shows people over 70 within weeks of weight training are as strong as 20 year olds. So throw the idea of "Aging = Body falling apart" out, it's not a productive thought pattern and it's a lie!*

My Objectives for You in This Book Are:

1) Show you all the benefits (financial, personal, social) that huge vital energy bring you.

2) To understand how to easily and quickly choose exercise and diet wisely to maximize and optimize your vitality *no matter what level of health you are at right now.*

3) Develop a healthy respect and understanding of basic health principles and how your body works (I warn you here, many will run contrary to popular wisdom).

4) Show you the foods and exercises that work and those that you should avoid at all costs.

5) Give you the tools to live healthily every day and *never be afraid* of disease again.

6) Provide you with a 40 day Plan of Action to get healthy.

If I do this, I believe I will have succeeded and that feels good since I enjoy helping and sharing what works (and doesn't) with you. Enjoy the book and thank you for entrusting your interest in my ideas, your health and this book.

I believe in you, and you should believe in your ability to do this (Live an outrageously healthy vital life) and I will make it as easy as I possibly can to enjoy the process.

"The human body is the best picture of the human soul."
L. Wittgenstein

Bountiful Benefits To a Vital And Healthy Body

If you want to get healthy, you need incentives, "carrots" to motivate you. There will also be some "sticks", some of the information will frighten you. We often hear "without your health, you have nothing!" I agree, but few back up their words with actions. Of course you have your own reasons for wanting more health. I have listed below many of the reasons to want to be vibrant. I have discovered these through working with my clients over the years. Why should you want to be healthy?

Energy is the currency of life. Without it you literally have nothing!

As a good summary here are the areas having huge vitality and health will *create a better and longer life.*

1. **Family:** More energy to play, connect and be with your kids, not being dead-tired after work. Better connection through more attention to each moment.

2. **Significant Other:** More quality time for connecting, laughing as well as an improved and much more satisfying sex life will benefit you and your significant other. I can tell you from personal experience, as my girlfriend is a personal trainer: we have a sex life most 20 year olds would envy both in quality, quantity and joy. *Do not underestimate the power of health on your sexual proficiency, appetite and enjoyment.* An

important piece of advice here: If only one partner becomes vital and healthy and the other does not, disconnections occur which can and often do break couples apart. *So, do this as a couple.* If your partner does not support your drive to a healthier more vital life you may want to re-evaluate the relationship as your health should be your number 1 priority no matter what or who is there (this may sound radical, but so is cancer).

3. **Fun:** What do you do for fun? If you are not in peak health the odds are high that you don't enjoy the same variety and intensity of activities you did in your early 20's when anything was possible. You have also probably bought into the "no one (sane) over X years old does that!" insanity our society propagates. I personally, still ride a dirt bike, jump off small cliffs skiing, snowboard, climb trees, dive from high places, and roughhouse with the kids, run in the woods with my dog, etc. Have you skydived yet? I haven't but plan to next summer. I can tell you how fun and liberating it is to wear clothes the same size I did in university (20 years ago)!

4. **Money:** A few years ago before my health transformation, I could barely handle my full time job and had little energy for anything else. Today, I do that job, run 2 companies, am writing this book and have plans for hundreds of other things. Without the huge energy I enjoy daily this would be impossible. Think about it, what could you do with an extra quality 3 to 5 hours a day? I'll bet you, you could make a lot more money! By living healthier you will live longer and have more opportunities for an inheritance. *Money is worthless without the energy and health to use it.* Ask anyone in a long term care health facility, and take in the movie "The Bucket List".[3]

5. **Personal Development:** What classes, courses have you been wanting to take but just can't muster the energy and willpower to do so. Salsa lessons, self improvement classes and martial arts. Weekend seminars to grow. Travelling is so enjoyable when you have limitless energy to explore, visit and

see new things. Being able to focus better and longer before tiring while reading a book allows more growth in all other aspects of your life.

6. **<u>Career</u>:** How much more dynamic would you be in the office, in sales or whatever it is you do if you were always there, really there? A lot more! And you would enjoy it more. You could get promoted faster to better positions. It is a fact slimmer/ healthier (more vital) people are seen as more industrious and enjoy more career promotions.

"To lose one's health renders science null, art inglorious, strength unvailing, wealth useless, and eloquence powerless."
Herophilus C. 300 B.C.

1.2   Remarkable Regeneration

The Human Body is Powerful, Self Regulating and self-repairing, *given it has the right materials to do what it was meant to do!*

How often does the human heart beat in one day? Let's calculate: 70 beats per minute * 60 minutes * 24 hours = over 100,000 beats per day! It pumps thousands of liters (hundreds of gallons) of blood every day. Did you know your nose can discriminate over 10,000 smells!

The aging body is often compared to an aging car. This is a ridiculous comparison. How many cars do you know that filter, change and renew their oil supply? How many cars, repaint themselves overnight when rocks damaged the paint? How many cars get faster and more resistant the harder you push them? How many cars become more efficient and able to resist environmental challenges better as they age? If you know of one car like this, I will buy this magical manufacturing company and make millions immediately! How many cars will clean and get rid of huge particles that were not made to go in your gas tank? *Your body does all these things and more every day!* Yet most of us treat our body as if it was an invincible tank we should throw as much garbage into to see what it can take before breaking. Then we complain that "it's normal, I'm aging!" You are aging, but the decrease in health is due to the accumulation of poisons/toxins you and the environment have continually put in it over the course of your life (and continue to introduce daily).

"No citizen has a right to be an amateur in the matter of physical training….what a disgrace it is for a man to grow old without ever seeing the beauty and strength of which his body is capable."

Socrates

1.3   *What Is Health?*

Most people *erroneously* believe health is the absence of disease. This is not a satisfactory or sustainable definition as a body free of disease can still lack vitality, energy and spark. Health is vibrant, almost unlimited energy, vitality constantly allowing you to do, think, create whatever you want (this is my definition!).

Some Other Popular Definitions of Health:

1. Optimal human fulfillment and productivity equaling quality of life.

2. Health is a state of complete physical, mental or social well-being and not merely the absence of infirmity.

3. Health is the result individual responsibility – choosing healthy over non-healthy.

__Key Health tip #1__ : You control the quality of your health: Step up and take control or someone with different goals will drive you down a path (of illness) you probably won't like (they are simply preaching for their choir!). Take the reins of your health now!

1.4 <u>Meaningful Mindset Maximizes Health</u>

The number one (#1) predictor or indicator of success in anything is mindset or psychology. Your health mindset is the most important predictor of your health for it determines how you see food, exercise, sleep, stress, etc. What are some of your traditional thoughts around health (both positive and negative?). I will cover emotions and mindset in more detail later. More relevant though: *Are these thoughts helpful or hurtful to you?* Are they based on true facts, hearsay or common sense? I'll bet *most of what we learn around health is via advertising, school, doctors, friends and family.* Here's the problem: Many of these sources don't have the latest information. Another interesting distinction is that *we often seek health from those who have not achieved it themselves!* I for one would rather listen to those who are successful, living healthily now.

I don't say I have the end all be all as information continuously comes out which change the game and the rules. However, I have looked around as of late early 2009 and new ideas really bring a new reality to traditionally limiting thinking around health. Again I urge you to suspend your critique and *use common sense when evaluating all I say to you! Better yet: try it in your own body and see/feel/experience for yourself.* Remember, Christopher Columbus was ridiculed when he said the world was spherical, not flat. Blood letting used to be thought to eliminate evil spirits. We used to think smoking was acceptable. Need any more? *So again I beg for your own health, use common sense and keep an open mind, no matter how strong the urge to discount these ideas as "vegetarian insanity" or "environmental fascism", etc.* Your body and I thank you in advance!

1.5   *Fact Or Fiction (Common Myths)*

Some common traditional beliefs around health/food:

"We must eat 3 meals a day from the 4 food groups"

"Vegetarians are weak and lack protein."

"Starve a cold, feed a fever!"

"Chicken Soup is good for a cold"

"As you get older, your body falls apart; energy and all capacities decrease dramatically"

"Milk is a great source of calcium"

"You need to eat meat/dairy to get protein"

"You need to minimize fat in your diet!"

"Diet pop is better than sugared pop"

"Working out hard gets better results."

"Coffee is good for you and keeps you focused and sharp."

"Alcohol, especially wine is good for you."

"You can catch all kinds of nasty colds and you should run to get your flu shot every year".

Fitness is the same as health.

I will cover each of these later in greater detail. *They are all FALSE.*

"Tell me what you eat, and I will tell you what you are."
                                    Anthelme Brillat-Savarin
                                    The Physiology of Taste

1.6 *Basic Cell Biology*

If you ask most people, "*Where does energy in your body come from?*" Most people will tell you they get energy from food. This is only partially true. Vital energy in the human body comes from the energy produced in individual cells.

Your quality of health and life is simply the quality of the life of your cells!

Energy is the building block of life. It makes all our opportunities available to us, it can be likened to human "fuel". Think about it. If you're financially wealthy but sickly…will you enjoy life? Not very likely! Without energy we have no life. Unfortunately most of us worry more about the energy requirements of our car or house! We need to begin looking at the most important energy of all: the one propelling, sustaining us and allowing us to enjoy ALL life has to offer. Most people become financially successful in a direct proportion to their health and energy decreasing, a real shame.

All cells have a job to do. Nerve cells carry electric impulses, stomach cells absorb food, red blood cells carry oxygen, etc. There are between 10 to 100 trillion cells in your body!

Each cell is an individual or organism that can be analyzed through a process called The Krebs (or Citric Acid) Cycle, energy is produced.

"The Krebs cycle refers specifically to a complex series of chemical reactions in all cells that utilize oxygen as part of their respiration process."[4]

Energy is the currency of life. Cells as with all living things need 3 critical ingredients to survive and thrive:

1) **Oxygen**
2) **Water**
3) **Ability to eliminate waste**

1) Oxygen is the main source of energy in all living cells and the body. This energy drives the metabolic processes in the body. These are absorption, digestion, waste elimination, respiration and circulation. A lack of oxygen destroys cells. Without oxygen, some cells die, others *mutate* into other anaerobic versions, an example being cancer. Cells removed from animals (mammals such as rats) deprived of oxygen once reinserted create cancer. As a matter of fact, if given basic needs, cells can live forever! Who knew!

<u>*What causes cells to die?*</u>

According to Dr. Stanley Robbins of Harvard Medical School there are 6 causes of cell atrophy (dying).

1) Decreased Oxygen workload
2) Enervation (stress)
3) Diminished blood supply
4) Inadequate nutrition
5) Loss of endocrine stimulation
6) Aging

2) Water is the most abundant substance in the body. Common Sense tells us the earth is 70% + water. The human body is 70-80% water; the cells have the exact same makeup. Water is used in cells to breakdown other materials, it helps carry out chemical reactions. It also diffuses and moves substances.

3) Lastly, and often ignored is the ability for a cell to *eliminate and excrete (get rid of its waste through normal means such as sweat, urination and defecation) its cellular waste.*

2   Critical Circulatory Systems:

1. Blood is the primary medium that delivers oxygen and nutrients to the body. Blood is literally the river of life. It is the transportation medium for oxygen and nutrients to the body's cells and tissues and it eliminates waste. A typical adult has 7 liters (almost 2 gallons of blood).

2. The primary system of eliminating wastes is the lymph system. It cleans and returns tissue fluid to the blood and destroys toxins that enter the body. *A little known fact is that your body has 300% more lymph fluid than blood, or 22+ liters.* The lymphatic system brings disease- fighting materials to cells, take dead germs away and supplies protein filled plasma back to the heart. When this system is blocked we become defenseless against all manner of foreign invaders such as viruses, fungi and bacteria. This happens in two ways, a) nourishment can't reach cells and b) infection fighting material doesn't get to the cells! 3 things keep this system clean. A) Vital and life-giving nutrients, B) Oxygen-rich water and most critically C) deep diaphragmatic breath.

1.7   The True Source of Aging and Disease

The True Source of Aging and Disease is not Physical age! As mentioned earlier our bodies are incredibly powerful self-maintaining machines that can handle anything when in its healthy (and normal) state. The primary overwhelming cause of our illnesses is predominantly: *the accumulation of toxins in the body's bloodstream.* Our bodies are designed to eliminate poisonous toxins from our bloodstream. Dr. Isaac Jennings (founder of The Philosophy of Natural Hygiene) said that the cause of an individual disease may be caused by a given circumstance (virus, etc.). The *primary source* of the problem is those activities that decrease the amount of life force in our bodies!

"Dr Isaac Jennings (of Oberlin, Ohio, USA) who, after practicing medicine for 20 years, began to ask questions when, during a fever outbreak in the summer of 1815, a patient who rested, drank water and did nothing, recovered in absolute record time compared to patients who had been medicated. Based on this, Dr Jennings noted similar results with many other patients."[5]

Our life forces are depleted by the fact we (21st century "civilized" humans) eat foods that *require more nerve energy to digest than they produce in the cells.* This causes a constant and increasing deficit (along with free radicals created by emotional stress) which cause disease. Predictably, Dr. Jennings was widely attacked by "traditional" doctors.

The following is in support of the flu or cold *being the body's cure:*

"The symptoms of fever, runny nose, etc. are created by the body's immune response to both inhibit the growth and spread of the microbes to flush the toxins from the system and clean up the environment so there is no more breeding ground. So, the goal is to help the body detoxify and flush the irritation. The faster this happens, the sooner you will be well."[6]

We do this (get rid of the toxins and waste) by drinking copious amounts of water and *not by putting artificial chemicals that your body needs to eliminate in addition to the cold!*

Are you sitting down? If not please do, this is *huge!* Remember keep an open mind!

Disease is the body's attempt to cure itself. Disease is the cure!

"All truth goes through 3 steps: 1st it is ridiculed. 2nd it is violently opposed. Finally it is accepted as self-evident."

A. Schopenhaur

The body's response to this lowered nerve energy and decreased efficiency (functional) is the *elimination* of toxins from the system. There are 4 ways toxins are eliminated:

a) The skin
b) The Respiratory system (lungs)
c) Bowels
d) Urinary tract

Key health tip 2: **Low energy people have reduced elimination! They don't eliminate well. As a reference, Healthy human bodies excrete (minimum) after every meal. How often do you go eliminate fecal matter? If it's once every day or once every 2 days. Your body is toxic!**

What are the causes for poisons toxins to build in the bloodstream?

1. *Eating more food than you can eliminate.* With reduced nerve energy in the body, the body never catches up. Take a break in eating, fast (liquids only) for a day or two if this occurs.

2. *Biochemical additives* and waste as well as animal products, i.e. substances your body can't use.

3. *An overly acidic diet.* This encourages micro-organisms (yeasts, molds, funguses, etc.) within your bloodstream to proliferate. They need to eat and they create waste on top of your unmoved waste! This adds to the toxicity of your system. I was sitting next to a woman at a seminar last weekend. Her breath reeked

of acidity. Her skin also looked very unhealthy. Common sense moment here: do you really think the human body was made to drink soft drinks, coffee (both pure acid), to eat acid forming foods such as fried foods, hydrogenated oils? Not on your life!

I have heard from a few sources in my research that it takes approximately 20 glasses of water to bring your body back to normal Ph after only 1 coffee or soft drink! Coffee, lifts your toxic body up? Yes it does *because your body is reacting to being poisoned and is stepping up its alert to rid your body of what it considers poisonous. Always recall: the body will do whatever it takes to survive!* After years of coffee, it takes more and more of it (as with any drug) to obtain effect and destroy your adrenal glands which stop working. *If you eliminate the acid, you won't need coffee!*

"Natural Forces within us are the true healers of disease."
Hippocrates

We are so out of balance, we are in a healing crisis. Our bodies can't heal themselves any more! Acne, colds and athlete's foot are great examples of your body trying to rid itself of toxins. What do we do? Most people take an artificial, toxic and chemically alien product that stops their body from healing itself. This slows down the body's natural ability and processes that help it cleanse and detoxify and add a greater strain on it.

The cause of your pain is rarely the source of your pain! What this means is that if you are experiencing symptoms, ensure you target the cause of the symptom otherwise you will keep getting other related ailments. This is the problem with mainstream healthcare, the source of the problem is rarely addressed, just the symptoms.

> *Key Health Tip #3: Let your body do its work to get rid of whatever ailment it has. Don't medicate the condition other than drinking large quantities of water and eating high water content foods.*

1.8   *Poisonous Pathways*

When your body (via the bloodstream) is poisoned by your lifestyle, your bloodstream becomes acidic (ugly scene here: *your body is rotting from the inside out*). How did you get poisoned? There are a few pathways most of us take to this poisoned state. These are:

A) Food that was inundated with very nasty micro-organisms (examples such as Escherichia coli, Clostridium Difficile).

B) The food eaten was already in the process of decay (animal flesh)

C) Foods were improperly combined causing them to ferment and putrefy (rot) in your digestive system.

D) Improper breathing, full diaphragmatic breathing was limited (due to stress)

E) Creation of anaerobic condition in blood system

The following are some of the clearest symptoms that your bloodstream is toxic and poisonous. I've listed them from mildly annoying to extremely dangerous. Remember: Your body never lies!

Mildly annoying	Phlegm, gas, perspiration, burping, heartburn
Unpleasant	Constipation, trouble sleeping, cough, headaches, cramps,
	low energy,
Painful	Joint pain, diarrhea, vomit, rash, skin eruptions,
Extremely Dangerous	Fever, heart rate increase/decrease, kidney, urinary problems, irregular breathing

As you can see, all the above are common conditions most people take for granted or don't worry about, i.e. most people are poisoned and this causes many of the ailments above!!

21

1.9 *Disease Destinations Demystified*

Top 10 Killers in The United States (Jan. 2007):[7]		
RANK	**CAUSE OF DEATH**	**NUMBER**
1	Heart Disease	727,000
2	Cancer	540,000
3	Cerebrovascular (e.g. Stroke)	160,000
4	Pulmonary Diseases	109,000
5	Accidents and Injuries	96,000
6	Pneumonia & Influenza	87,000
7	Diabetes	63,000
8	Suicide	31,000
9	Kidney Disease	26,000
10	Liver Disease	25,000

Do you notice a pattern above? Fully 8 out of 10 are diet-related! Only suicide and Accidents are *not* diet and lifestyle related. An argument could even be made that suicide is aided by depression which can be alleviated greatly by being healthier.

A really simple way to understand disease (and alternatively → health!) is the following.

Disease occurs and is created when more tearing down of your system is happening than building up!

Doesn't this make extreme common sense? When the body is in a weakened state caused by the above-mentioned poisoning, there is a deficiency or diminishment of life energy or force.

> **_Key health Tip #4_**: *Disease can only be created by us (via lifestyle) when more tearing down of your system is happening than building up (via proper foods and activity)! Otherwise, perfect health!*

1.91   *Major Misinformation Mix-up*

Who invented astrology? Some may say Galileo, it was invented before Christ. It used to be of the same branch as astronomy. In the 16th century they separated and became two sciences. In history, it is widely accepted that Christopher Columbus discovered America. This is an "urban myth". The Vikings via Leif Ericksson landed in Newfoundland in the year 1000, some 492 years before Columbus.

In biology a similar misconnection has occurred. Louis Pasteur's Germ Theory postulated that outside (in the world) germs invade our bodies and cause disease. Interestingly, it turns out Pasteur was a plagiarist (and much better marketer!) who stole and warped Mr. Pierre Bechamp's ideas. *Bechamp proved germs existed 6 years earlier.* That was the least of the problem. Pasteur *misinterpreted Bechamp's theory* and admitted so on his deathbed. What was more important than the germ was the environment (terrain) the germs entered! Pasteur admitted: "The microbe is nothing, the terrain is everything."[8]

Unfortunately, most people still believe they can "catch" an infection or cold. What a costly misunderstanding.

"Your range of available choices – right now – is limitless."
C. Frederick

One of the major problems with so-called "general knowledge" around health is a mistaken or erroneous source, cause, result relationship.

Source → Cause → Result relationship.

As mentioned earlier, most of us (including many uninformed in the medical profession) are targeting the wrong things in our search for causes of disease.

Here is an analogy. Suppose there is a problem in your house with termites. The termites are attracted and encouraged by old, rotting wood left untreated (which they eat and digest via special bacteria which break down cellulose).

"Entomologists (insect biologists) have discovered that termites are attracted to one percent carbon dioxide, which is the exact amount given off by rotting wood."[9]

You call in the exterminators immediately and the termites are all killed. Unfortunately the brittle untreated wood remains. The termites return after a period. And do so over and over again and again. Unless the cause of the attraction (the rotting wood) is rectified or removed, problems will continue and get worse.

Our bodies are rotting (due to the toxins and wastes created by our acid lifestyle), and are similar to untreated (low immune function in humans) wood. The termites in our body are germs, bacteria and viruses causing disease. We must get our wood (bodies) in peak condition or deal with the termites (get rid of the rot = acid life)! If not, the house of our health will crumble and be destroyed (disease and death).

What is wonderful is that the medical community is now teaching more recently updated material than it used to. Many older, traditional medical practitioners are unaware or unwilling to adjust to or learn this new information. Thankfully there are many alternative health care professionals who understand this, including naturopaths and osteopaths. Ensure your health practitioner is aware.

"The concept, however of one etiologic agent to one disease – developed from the study of infections or single-gene disorders – *is no longer sufficient.* Genetic factors are clearly involved in some of the common environmentally induced maladies, such as atherosclerosis and cancer, and the environment may also have *profound influences* on certain genetic diseases.[10]

So again, *disease does not attack healthy systems or cells.* When we keep our cells healthy we are healthy and energetic and can live without fear and free of health-related worry! That's phenomenal news deserving celebration!

Koch's Postulates

The Classical criteria for determining if disease is infectious and caused by a specific microbe are called Koch's Postulates (named for Nobel Prize laureate Robert Koch) in the last century. This work is still the scientific basis against every disease is evaluated.

The bottom line here is that *germs are not found in every case of disease.* And some forms of the disease occurred without exposure to the germ! *This means that germs do not equal disease.*

A great example of this is that the Herpes Simplex (HSV) virus is at any given time, carried by almost 75% of all people – most people never have or ever will experience any symptoms of HSV.

Perfectly healthy people carry the germs of diphtheria, pneumonia, tuberculosis, etc. These people do not have, never did and won't develop these diseases if they remain at a low toxicity level. Here is another piece of information disproving the "germs produce disease" argument. Germs do not "attack and/or destroy" healthy tissue. No germs *have ever and will never* multiply in normal healthy cells and tissue. Germ theory is unsupportable. Many attempts have been made to inject the flu virus into the bloodstream, into the throats and on the food of healthy navy personnel. No appreciable reactions occurred.

> *__Key Health Tip #5:__ When healthy, the human body has no chance of being "invaded" or "attacked" by viruses, bacteria or other living pathogens. The body's natural defenses are just too strong!*

2.0 *Foolish Flu Falsehoods*

Every fall like clockwork we begin hearing about the latest "flu bug". These "bugs" usually have exotic, obscure and scary sounding names (to scare you into getting a flu shot) such as the Shanghai, Hong Kong, Bird and now Swine Flu. Every fall we are warned to get our flu shots to "protect" against the upcoming possible yet probable misery of the flu. Most of these articles are published and created by the pharmaceutical giants who create the flu vaccine and sell it!

I believe the flu vaccine *does not work, I'll let you make your own decisions and deductions* but here is some food for thought:

- It is believed that more than 60% of health professionals choose not to get the flu vaccine *even though it's free and they are "at risk". If professionals don't believe in it why should we?*

- The vaccine is created with the last year's flu remnants so it can be ready for sale on time for fall (the dangerous "flu season") to maximize profits. No one even knows if they will work for this year!

- The vaccine is made of chicken cells which contain huge amounts of pathogens

Many of these flu shots contain Mercury as part of the preservative thimerosol, a known neurotoxin, and it is still in some vaccines. If you must get a shot, request a thimerosol-free vaccine. *The evidence shows that flu vaccines have little or no effect.* There is little comparative evidence that the vaccines are safe. I can tell you that personally I do not take flu vaccines because I have serious reservations about the *long-term neurological effects.* A tremendous amount of medical literature states that *just because you get a flu vaccine doesn't mean you won't get the flu.* I have not had the flu shot in 5 years and have never been healthier.

The *British Medical Journal* looked at all the research behind flu shots and came up with some interesting conclusions.

- The evidence shows that *flu vaccines have little or no effect.*

- There is little comparative evidence that the vaccines are safe.

- The authors noted a "gap" between guidelines that call for mass vaccination and the evidence to support those guidelines.

There are a significant number of people who get quite ill immediately after receiving the flu vaccine. So, say no to the *flu vaccine if you want to stay healthy!*

Let's use our common sense again. *When does the flu season start?* Late fall or early winter, season peaks in early January. What's convenient about that is it mirrors the Thanksgiving to New Year's yearly celebrations. Stress, overeating, drinking and people generally breaking their normal routines of food and exercise occur at that same time of year. *Most people eat horribly large, dead meals in this period, they don't get enough rest and they over-indulge in alcohol.* All these conditions point to a decreased immunity function over the holiday season leading to the "explosion" in flu cases.

Key Health Tip #6 The Holidays' overeating, drinking and stress dramatically increase the likelihood of our bodies being a fertile ground for all viruses including the flu.

Most people worry more about their spring wardrobe than their food and drink habits.

A personal painful and telling experiment: I was involved in a little experiment recently (it didn't start out that way but as with most things in life it just happened!) but it did reprove to myself how good I was feeling really was linked to the food changes I had made. The night before I had one ounce of dark rum in orange juice with popcorn at home. The next day, dehydrated with a headache. I went for a so called "normal" Sunday restaurant breakfast. I started out with coffee as most people do. I then ordered the big breakfast. A combination of 3 eggs sunny side up, bacon, whole wheat toast (no butter), 1.5 pancakes with maple syrup and an orange juice.

Well let me tell you! The results were quite conclusive. I tried having 3 glasses of water after to somehow rebalance after this unusual and cruel punishment (to my pretty freshly somewhat well-balanced system). Within 2 hours I had a massive energy drain, I just wanted to sleep. I was burping up the food, my stomach felt bloated and queasy. My breath was rank and smelled of something dead. It was reminiscent of that movie "Supersize me" where the gentleman goes on a fast food month-long binge that ends up becoming a serious threat to his life. So even if I had one of these types of breakfasts a week it would seriously throw off my energy and healthy balance. *Just because you may not be feeling this way after this type of breakfast is a Great indicator how acid you are, your body is used to low energy food! This should scare you!* You should immediately run to the drugstore and buy the cheapest indicator of health ever invented: the pH strip. I went home and tested my urine's pH, as expected it was down to 5. which is acidic (optimal is 6 to 6.5). See section 3.4 on Alkalinity.

As background information, for the last 16 years I have always had a giant mixture of 7-10 fruits blended with yogurt in a blender (or fresh fruit and dried fruit when on trips) in the morning. To imagine adding burgers, pizza, cigarettes, alcohol, fried foods, coffee was unthinkable and really quite frightening. I'm feeling nauseated as I write this! I can report that even a day after the impacts of the food continued, from stomach pain, bloated feeling and gaseousness. Again if you don't feel this way after these meals, your body is probably already toxic. This will cause you to get very tired quickly.

3.0 *Velocity to Vitality and High Health*

Now that you understand some of the basic biology, let's get into what works. Let's learn how to implement it into your life in a way that works, a way that will not be so painful that you don't stick to it. The following ideas or guidelines are the cornerstones of this work. If you implement the following simple ideas for the next 40 days, you will feel so good, you will never want to go back, guaranteed. The level of energy, strength, vitality you will feel, experience and enjoy will make you feel as if you were asleep your whole life. Everything will change, your nails will grow stronger, your breath better, your skin will require very little as it will be healthy, I can guarantee you won't need (or even desire) coffee, pop or other stimulants. You will be frisky as if you were 18 again. Your mind will be clearer, you will sleep better, eliminate better, sweat nice, etc.

Here is an overview of the path I will take to get you to incredible vitality, energy and health. I will use the analogy of The Diamonds (great things improving your health) and Dinosores (destroyers of health).

8 Health Diamonds

1. Breathing & Lymphasizing

2. Living Water & Foods

3. Essential Oils

4. Alkalinity

5. Aerobic Energy

6. Peak Nutrition

7. Alignment/Power

8. Mindset

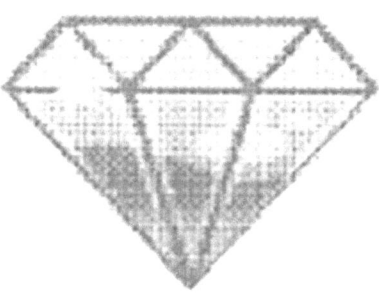

The 4 Dinosores (Destroyers) of Health

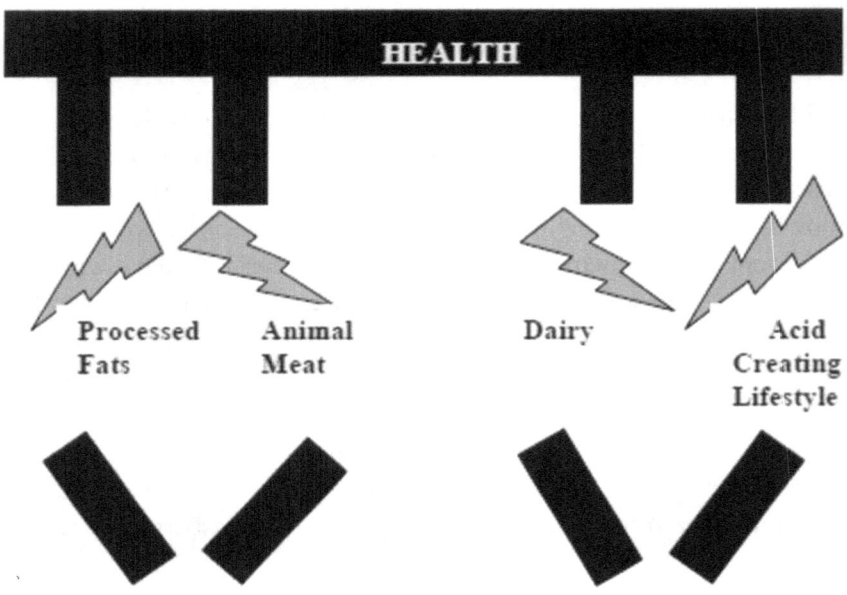

Processed Fats

Animal Meat

Dairy

Acid Creating Lifestyle

3.1 *1ST Diamond: Beneficial Breathing And Life-Giving Lymphasizing*

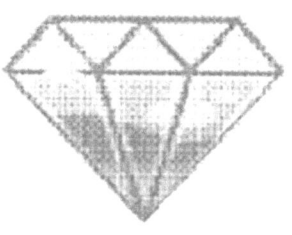

3.11 *Breathing:*

We don't know how to breathe! The most important piece of the puzzle of our health as humans is Oxygen. Human life could not exist without it. Oxygen is moved through blood to our cells where it is used in cells to fuel them and energy via Adenosine Triphosphate (ATP, the Krebs cycle I described earlier). Water is 1/3 Oxygen (H2O). How long can a human live without food? Most people die after 30 days. How long without Water? Maximum, two or three days. *Oxygen, 6 to 9 minutes!* So Oxygen's importance is critical.

"There is no single more powerful- or more simple – daily practice to further your health and well being than breathwork." [11]

Suggestions around breathing:

1. Breathe in slowly on a count to 12, hold your breath 8 seconds then let it out slowly to a count of 12. Repeat for 20 breaths morning and evening.

2. Most of us walk around holding our chests up so we look like we don't have a tummy or gut. Look at your pets breathe, they don't breathe from their chests! *Proper breathing is from the diaphragm.* The lungs are larger on the bottom than top so by breathing from our chests we lose 50% of our lung capacity.

3. Laughing, smoking and yawning all get much larger amounts of oxygen into our lungs. This is one of the reasons many people smoke! Why not learn the proper way and use it consistently?!

3.12 *Lymphasizing*

As previously mentioned, our lymphatic system is 200% larger than our blood system. So elimination must be very important. We need to get the cellular waste out quickly and efficiently. What follows are some suggestions to successfully lymphasize.

1. Breathing per above helps lymphasize via diaphragmatic pressure on the lymphatic system.

2. Buy and use a small trampoline (also called a rebounder) 10 minutes in the morning. This has *multiple* benefits including up and down motions (cleanse cells), strengthen the cells membranes like a resistance workout for your cells. Improves posture, muscle tone, coordination, balance, rhythm and increase your energy. Help maximize heart muscle efficiency. Most importantly it accelerates the elimination of all wastes via your huge lymphatic drainage system.

"The Art of Lymphology as a holistic lifestyle was created by Dr Samuel E West. It is the practice of moving the lymph by gently bouncing on a trampoline and involves correct breathing, correct body movement, proper diet and positive thought patterns. As we get the lymphatic system circulating, we are converting mechanical energy into electrical energy to literally "turn the body back on".

Lymphasizing is thought to free trapped blood proteins, remove lasting pain, and remove energy blockages and eliminate disease.

"A rebounder, or mini trampoline, allows you to stimulate and strengthen every cell in the body simultaneously...It is very effective for health and weight loss." [12]

You can use your rebounder while watching television, listening to your music. You don't have to bounce high at all, simply having your body leave the surface, rise, stop and return is enough! I strongly assert this is the single most important piece of exercise equipment everyone should own.

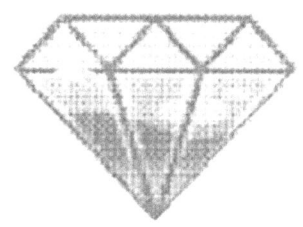

3.2   2ⁿᵈ Diamond
Live Waters And Living
Fresh Foods

Even if you ignore every tip in this book (I quite hope and doubt you will) this next subject will allow a huge change. The planet earth is covered by over 70% water. Water is an essential and crucial component of *all living matter*. Here are some other key statistics around optimal water content of human tissues:

Human Brain →	76% water
Human Lungs →	90% water
Human Blood →	83+% water
Human Blood Plasma →	98% water
Human Bones →	25% water

See a pattern here? Even bones have 25% water to stay flexible!

"Drink more water" is mentioned so much we *underestimate its critical nature.* Life-giving, non-negotiable processes such as circulation, excretion and *digestion can not occur without it!* It carries nutrients to all critical body substances, plays a cornerstone role in temperature regulation and (you may not know this one) is used as a building material for growth and repair of the cells in your body.

Did you know that you can't live more than 10 days without water? *You can only lose 10% of your body's water and still survive. The hard fact here:* Most of us check our oil level in our car much more often than our own hydration levels! Insanity!!!

"Water is the mother of the vine, the nurse of the fountain of fecundity, the adorner and refresher of the world."

Charles Mackay, The Dionysia

Dr. Ferrydoon Batmanghelidj [13] recounts treating over three thousand (3000) prisoners *with water only* (as medication was not available!). He drank water and noticed hunger pains go away. His brilliant book "Your Body's Many Cries for Water" labels many modern diseases as different stages of dehydration. *Water not only maintains health but can cure disease!*

Some of his findings include:

The body loses 2.5 liters of water per day. It is replaced by food and water. However, environmental conditions and exercise increase its needs drastically. Even mild dehydration causes decreased coordination, impaired judgment and fatigue. Side-effects include stress, headaches, back pain, allergies, weight gain, asthma, high blood pressure, and Alzheimer's disease. Before taking in a coffee or energy drink, drink 3 tall glasses of water, you won't need them (coffee or energy drinks) anymore. Before taking any pain relievers for a headache, drink two glasses of water.

1. *A dry mouth is the last outward sign of dehydration!* If you are thirsty you're cells are already dehydrated. *If you are thirsty it is said that you have already lost 4 to 5 cups of water!* Just a small amount of dehydration can cause a decrease in mental processing and acuity. Your attention and concentration can decrease by 13% and short term memory by 7% with mild dehydration (defined as a loss of 1% or more of body weight due to fluid losses).

2. *Thirst perception* decreases with age.

3. *A carefully hydrated body produces colorless urine!* A *somewhat dehydrated* body produced yellow urine. A *severely dehydrated body* produces orange or dark urine.

4. ***Water Removers*: Caffeine, Soda and Alcohol Kill You By Rotting You Out!**

All Alcohol (yes even wine!) *Halts* the process whereby water is allowed into cells! The "buzz" we get with one drink is caused by millions of our brain cells dying!

Caffeine stimulates the kidneys *to secrete more water out of the body* than there is water in the coffee in the first place. Do you know what the "high" you feel when you drink coffee is? Are you sitting for this? *Your Body is actually on high alert mobilizing to remove the poison you just willingly put into it.* After years of this abuse, your adrenal glands slow down and you need more and more of it. Did you know that scientists are just now discovering and proving *that one of the primary causes of breast cancer in women is coffee?* It makes sense because breast tissue is fatty and this is where poisonous acids such as caffeine are going to be brought to be surrounded by fat cells. You should be aware that the body in its incessant will to survive will move *all dangerous substances (toxins) as far as possible from its vital organs.* As with all other drugs it is addictive and has a medium and long-term massive negative impact on the body.

"Another ill effect of the drug-caffeine like all other traditional drugs is that with time, you need to increase your consumption in order to experience the same results despite of which the caffeine consumption does not provide you anymore with the desired lift. When the body reaches such a severe point, this condition is known as adrenal depletion."[14]

I will cover coffee in more detail later.

Soft Drinks are anything but "soft". They are acid and have huge sugar (or worse Aspartame) in them. Americans consume *64 Gallons (256 liters)* of soda per capita per year! The average American last year consumed *581 cans* of soda! Big Gulps are the equivalent of 5 -7 cans of drink.

We will discuss soft drinks in more detail later as well.

"Water is the most neglected nutrient in your diet but one of the most vital."

Kelly Barton

Easily Calculate the Quantity of Water You Should Drink Per Day:

> Here is the calculation: **Drink 50%** of your body weight in ounces a day.
>
> So in my case I weigh 165 lbs, so 83 ounces of water ➜ **2.47 Liters of water**

Ideally, you should never go more than 15 – 20 minutes without sipping water. Also start drinking water first thing in the morning, this is when your body is at its most toxic and dehydrated.

Always stop drinking water 30 minutes before eating!

6. For athletes: weigh yourself before and after a hard workout to see how much water you need. Overdrinking is not good for you.

7. Where to get Drinking Water:

Tap water is definitely a hit and miss affair. Old city pipes allow lead levels to get dangerously high. All municipalities have different systems and ways of verifying their water. Most municipalities use Chlorine, Fluorine or Bromine. Both these substances do kill parasites but also are toxic to the human body.

"It (tap water) contains dissolved iron and manganese, calcium salts and magnesium that lead to wear and tear of the plumbing equipment and bathroom accessories. The water does damage to the human body too. On the one hand, chlorine (added in water) kills most dangerous microbes. On the other hand, it is one of the causes of atherosclerosis. Besides, chlorine forms carcinogenic substances when it mixes with organic matter present in water."[15]

Most bottled water is simply tap water put through a few filters to have it taste better. This industry is unregulated by the FDA! Anecdotal evidence recommends waters which come from foreign deep wells, do your research. Reverse osmosis seems to be the defacto best way to filter water. It removes most foreign elements (including chlorine, fluorine, chemicals, pesticides, heavy metals, bacteria and viruses). You can talk to your local health food store or the search the internet.

A Quick Test

Just for your own curiosity, try this test to determine how much water and live food *you are eating/ drinking.*

Write down everything that has passed through your lips in the last 24 hours. Don't cheat! Count gum, candy, chocolate, alcohol, coffee, cigarettes, drugs. (These are actually *"reverse" wa*ter, they dehydrate your body). If you are like most people, you had around 15% to 25% water-rich foods (fruits, vegetables, water). *The target is 70%!* This allows your body to cleanse itself. Failing this test means you are clogging your system gradually until it falls apart and fails (traditional "disease and aging" idea).

<hr>

__Key Health Tip #7:__ Every time you eat/drink ask yourself the following question. "Will this food cleanse me or clog me?". This removes the justifications many of us resort to.

<hr>

Terrifying! The typical average North American diet consists of only 15% water-rich foods.

This is literally equivalent to slow (it can get really quick too!) suicide! You might as well simply play Russian roulette with 4 bullets in the gun! These bullets can be cancer, arthrosclerosis, diabetes and Asthma. The following chart clearly shows the water content of common foods. The highest water contents are obviously the raw fruits and vegetables followed by meat then highly processed foods at the bottom with low or no energy. Note the seemingly decent water content of hamburger and eggs, but, these are never eaten raw.[16] I have reclassified the chart into food groups for better clarity.

Assorted Food's Water Content

FRUIT		VEGETABLES		MEAT	
Watermelon	93%	Squash Boiled	96%	Eggs Raw Whole	74%
Tomatoes Raw	93%	Cucumbers Raw	96%	Chicken Broiled	71%
Cantaloupe	91%	Lettuce Head	96%	Turkey Roasted	62%
Strawberries Raw	90%	Radishes Raw	95%	Veal Broiled	60%
Peaches Raw	90%	Celery	94%	Beef Raw Hamburger 54%	
Papayas Raw	89%	Peppers Green	94%	Ham Smoked Cooked 54%	
Grapefruit Raw	88%	Swiss Chard	94%	Pork Chops Broiled	45%
Plums Raw	87%	Pickles Dill	93%	**CARBOHYDRATES**	
Oranges	86%	Sauerkraut Canned	93%	Spaghetti Cooked	72%
Apples	85%	Bean Sprouts	92%	Bread Whole Wheat	35%
Apricots	85%	Rutabagas Boiled	90%	**DAIRY**	
Pineapple Raw	85%	Spinach Raw	92%	Cheese American	37%
Pears Raw	82%	Eggplant Raw	92%	Margarine	20%
Grapes	82%	Cabbage Raw	92%	Butter	20%
Raspberries	81%	Broccoli	91%	**NUTS & OILS**	
Fruit Cocktail	80%	Okra Boiled	91%	Almonds	7%
Cherries raw	80%	Cauliflower	91%	Pecans	7%
Bananas	76%	Collards boiled	91%	Walnuts	4%
		Watercress Raw	90%	Peanut Butter	Trace
		Pumpkin Canned	90%	Shelled Peanuts	Trace
		Onions	89%	**ASSORTED**	
		Carrots Raw	88%	Honey	15%
		Kale	87%	Jams/Preserves	30%
		Parsley Raw	86%	Molasses	25%
		Potatoes Raw	85%		
		Peas Raw	81%		
		Olives	80%		
		Sweet Potatoes Boiled in Skin	71%		

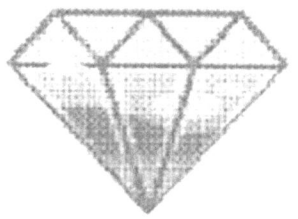

3.3   *3rd Diamond :*
Essential Oils

3.31   *Elemental Essential Oils*

As a modern society we have been taught that we must reduce/ eliminate *all fat* from our diets to lose weight, stay slim and maintain health. As with other bubbles I have been bursting, I've got a pin ready! We are inundated with *no-fat everything!* From cookies, chips, breads, etc. ad nauseum. Few people realize that *completely eliminating all the fat from your diet is the worst thing you can do!* A good rule of thumb is "if it is made by machine/man, don't eat it!"

The reality is that fats (natural ones of course) are critical to our proper functioning, the secret is to differentiate between *good, healthy fats and bad, unhealthy fats that kill!* Essential fatty acids are healing/ healthy fats. Did you know every cell in your body requires fats to function! For example, the human brain is made up of 60% fat!

Good fats are made up of essential fatty acids: Omega 3 & Omega 6. You must consume these fats to survive. Remove these fats and the critical lipid membrane around your cells begins to break down which is extremely hazardous to your health.

3.32   *Fabulous Fatty Acids: Opus of Optimal Health*

In the womb, the unborn child takes from its mother's body a substantial amount of the essential fats required to properly build its brain.

The *brain can not function without an adequate supply of essential fatty acids.* They are required for most of the vital functions in all cells, tissues and organ systems. They improve oxidation as well as metabolic rate. They transport minerals through the body. Fats help *energy* levels rise and increase stamina while decreasing recovery time!

Skin: Ladies (but men too!) especially here, why put chemical products, peels, creams which cost a fortune? These are like a coat of paint on a cracked foundation. Fatty acids create a smooth and velvety skin texture. Additionally, acne, psoriasis and eczema will be drastically reduced or disappear permanently! Also your sweat will be much less odorous. Instead of expensive creams and treatments, *consider nutrition as a remedy to keep wrinkles and other age-related issues away.* Studies have shown that eating whole grains, fruits, legumes, vegetables and omega-3 fatty acids can help keep skin healthy and youthful. Search out foods rich in lycopene, an antioxidant found in many red fruits and vegetables (good sources: tomatoes, watermelon and pink grapefruit). Also foods with beta-carotene, vitamin a (can be obtained in red, orange and yellow foods such as apricots, mango carrots and sweet potatoes). Vitamin B can be found in chick peas, mushrooms and lentils.

Digestion: Essential Fatty Acids help stop leaking intestines that can lead to auto-immune problems, allergies and inflammation (Irritable Bowel Syndrome).

The cardiovascular system uses fatty acids to transport cholesterol, lower triglycerides, make platelets less sticky and lower blood pressure. Fish oils have been proven to decrease cholesterol over 40% and triglycerides over 70% in certain studies.

Osteoarthritis and rheumatoid arthritis sufferers enjoy reduced inflammation.

Fatty Acids elevate *mood, lift depression, and improve our capacity to deal with pain and stress.* High stress levels promote high blood pressure, water retention, inflammation, and blood clot formation.

In the immune system, essential fatty acids *protect human DNA from different types of damage.* Although not a cure for cancer, they do benefit mammals and humans with cancer.

Obese and overweight people and animals can lose weight since their kidneys expel less water.

Deficiencies in Essential Fatty Acids include (but are not limited to):

Skin problems (eczema)	Slowed or sporadic child growth
Loss of hair	Liver problems
Dry Skin, Brittle nails, dry eyes	Kidney issues/ malfunctions
Cholesterol Rise	Fragile skin (water loss accompanied by thirst)
Sticky Platelets	Low energy levels with weakness
Glandular malfunction (increased infection risk)	Wounds heal slowly or not well at all.
Men stop producing testosterone → sterility	Miscarriages
Joint pain similar to arthritis	Irregular heartbeat
Tingling in limbs	Loss of motor skill coordination
Water retention	Tissue inflammation
Metabolic rate drops	Immune system failure

Now that we know why we need fats to become or stay healthy. Let's determine which fats we need.

3.33 *Fearsome (Bad) Fats*

Processed fats are fats that are broken down (destroyed) through cooking. As a matter of fact, *any cooking above 45 degrees Celsius (118 Fahrenheit) kills the fat and renders it unusable by the body.* Worse, it makes them toxic. Bad (Processed) fats cause poor circulation, high blood pressure, weak elimination, excess congestion as well as toxicity to the human body.

Processed = Bad = Killer Fats

- Most Margarines
- All animal fats such as Butter, cheese, eggs, Milk
- Vegetable oils (Wesson, Pam, Crisco)
- Shortening
- *Any and all deep fried foods, period!*

"The degenerative disease epidemic that wracks the nation came coincidentally with the introduction of engineered fats and oils. It is the type of fats and oils that we consume that is directly correlated to the rise of epidemic degenerative disease; it is not the amount of fats and oils that we eat that causes the problem."[17]

In my opinion, even more dangerous (because consumers believe they are safe) are the new "fat-free" products which use salt, sugar starches and chemicals and are devoid of life. To lose weight you need good fats (below) and avoid "bad fats". Also avoid sugar and "fat-free" products.

> *Key Health Tip #8: Avoid all Processed Fats (Animal fats and deep-fried foods) and all so-called "fat-free" foods. Increase your intake of unprocessed (naturally occurring) fats.*

3.34 *Great Life-Giving Fats*

When it comes to fats less is more, as in less processing. Unprocessed fats in their natural state support LUBRICATION of your entire system and the health of your whole body.

- **Flax Seed Oil** – Sprinkle on salads, pasta put in smoothie.

- **Olive Oil**. Put it in water when you cook whole wheat pasta, put on salads.

- **Avocado** – delicious in salads, Mexican food, shakes

- **Fish Oils** - Refrigerate after opening or get them in pill form. You want at least 800 mg EPA and 400 mg DHA. You want to get oils from non-toxic fish and/or lower in the food chain such as Krill Oil.

- **Nuts** such as Almonds, hazelnuts, pumpkin seeds and sunflower seeds. Here's a great trick, soak your almonds overnight in filtered water. They will become plump and tasty and increase their water content!

- **Udo's Oil** has the "accepted as optimal" 2:1 ratio of Omega 3's and Omega 6's. (Because too much of one will decrease the other). It is a mixture of other unrefined oils. You can mix this into a shake, on salad, or have it in a shot glass, etc. *it is not designed to be* a *cooking oil.* The recommended amount to take is 1 tablespoon per day per 22kg (50 lbs) body weight.[18]

Remember: Eskimos have the lowest rate of heart problems of any culture. *They eat tremendous amounts of fish oils and animal blubber from whales and seals.*

"Nothing will benefit human health and increase the chance of survival of life on Earth as much as the evolution to a vegetarian diet."

Albert Einstein

3.4   4ᵗʰ Diamond

Alkalinity : Great Greens

This book's main focus is to help you live your most vibrant healthy self, easily and quickly. It's about having a normal life while eating and feeling better than the masses. Remember, these are the same masses which have horrible track records on living well and long. When we are *not* at our top level health we are out of balance and get hit with low energy issues such as stress, fatigue, depression and disease. Balanced body chemistry and *maintaining the optimal ratio between acid and alkaline foods is critical to optimal health.* It is also an easy way to quickly check where you are at versus using the traditional weight scale or waist measurement which give you limited information. Our modern day lifestyles and diets *tend to acidity not alkalinity.* Too much acidity in your tissues and cells impact so many different systems it causes *all kinds of problems* such as lethargy, fatigue, obesity and in the medium or long term produces lifestyle-related deadly diseases such as cancer, stroke, heart disease, Diabetes, etc.

One of the most important issues, checks and balances your body presides over is to maintain alkalinity throughout your body to support cellular life. This level of alkalinity is maintained by all your systems such as breathing, circulation, digestion and hormonal production balance. These remove acid residues from your cells. The pH level (measure acid vs alkaline) in your body should *never deviate too far* on the acidic side (*common*) or too alkaline (*uncommon*). *If it deviates too far, cells are inundated and drown in their own toxic waste and die.*

The pH scale: Stands for Potential of hydrogen. Acids have a pH under 7 and alkalis a pH above 7. Right at 7 is neutral (neither acid or alkaline). The scale runs from 0 (pure acid…can burn through steel) to 14 (Pure alkaline).

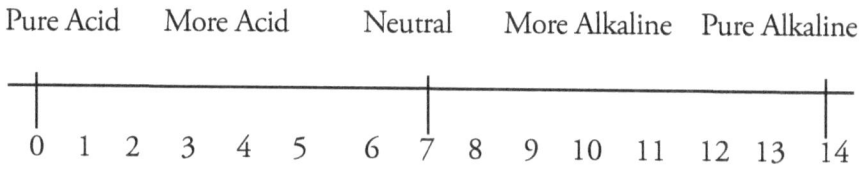

Pure Acid   More Acid   Neutral   More Alkaline Pure Alkaline

0 1 2 3 4 5 6 7 8 9 10 11 12 13 14

> **_Key Health Tip #9:_** *The cheapest health indicator you can buy is not a scale! It is pH strips available for at health food stores and some drugstores.*

Different body tissues maintain different levels of pH. The blood should be slightly alkaline, where urine, saliva and the digestive track should be slightly acid. The blood can not survive any major fluctuations in pH and still sustain life.

The most important aspect is the body's alkaline reserve (sodium bicarbonate) or Alkali Excess. Why? This reserve is stored until needed to neutralize excess acid in the body. If the body becomes acidic and depletes the alkaline reserve there is no buffer. Cells weaken and or die and this *is where your body functions become compromised, which leads to the creation of disease.* This is the number one thing you need to monitor to stay healthy: stay alkaline!

3.41   _Acidic pH : Body Blow_

There are numerous challenges to our bodies that are created and maintained by our modern acid lifestyle. Your lifestyle can be considered acid if you eat fried foods, all meats, dairy, drink pop, coffee, smoke, if you don't drink enough water or living foods, etc.

Here are the many common impacts of an acidic system.

1. A low (acid) pH allows cholesterol to bind to heavy metals and other debris increasing the rate *plaque builds up* in the vascular (blood) network (can lead to heart attack or stroke).

2. *Low Energy:* Your cells are inefficient and your metabolism drops making it harder to move!

3. Acid impairs electrolyte activity and increases the *likelihood of cellular mutations (otherwise known as cancer!).*

4. Acidosis disrupts lipid and fatty acid metabolism. This increases the arrival of neurological problems and imbalances in hormones within the endocrine system. This results in *urinary infections.*

5. The increased workload on the heart makes it *more difficult to control high blood pressure.*

6. Blood plasma when acidic acts as a chemical irritant that eats away at the smooth muscle inside the arteries and veins. This weakens the structural composition and creates irregular blood pressure. (requiring medications with huge side-effects).

7. The cell walls and membrane structures are damaged by free radicals. Consequences include *premature aging, eyesight and memory loss,* wrinkles, age spots, poor hormone regulation, etc.

8. Reduces oxygen affinity of hemoglobin in your blood. As we covered earlier oxygen depletion compromises all body functions.

9. *Most "overweight" people <u>do not</u> have a problem of "too-much fat",* *they have an acid problem!* Too much acid in the body creates two major challenges. A) It causes the body to produce more insulin which in turn signals the *body to store more fat!* And B) It causes the cells to break down due to constant pressure to produce more insulin. As noted many times the human body wants to survive at all costs! Your body stops dangerous acid from approaching all vital organs, it stores it in fat cells! Your body actually says "Hey, I want to live, let's make/retain some fat to surround this deadly acid!"

<u>Key Health Tip #10:</u> If you are overweight, you most likely have an acid problem. By becoming more alkaline, your body will get rid of the fat it used to surround the acid. Since it no longer needs to protect itself from acid, you shed weight as long as you stay alkaline!

3.42 *Easy and Fun Ways to Alkalize!*

Most important here is have fun, experiment, go gradually to allow your taste buds to adjust and really start tasting quality foods. Once your body loses its acidity, you will crave real and fresh food, and you will be able to taste all the intricacies in living food!

1. Put *lemon or lime* in the water you drink *all day*. Lemon and lime juice are both very alkaline, not acid as one would think.[19] Add some zest and gusto to your water with a bit of fresh mint.

2. Use *lemon* and a tiny amount of good salt (Himalayan or Celtic sea salt) for *salad dressing*. Most health food stores have recipes for salad dressing (flax seed oil, lemon juice, pepper and garlic make an interesting dressing).

3. Substitute *sprouted wheat breads* and pizza crusts for white or wheat.

4. Feed your need for texture and crunchiness! Often we crave textures which bad foods give us (chips, cookies and crackers). Baked tortilla chips with fresh guacamole. Crunchy veggies (carrots and celery) with hummus (chickpea spread). Sprouted wheat pita bread or tortillas with avocado, sun-dried tomato (adds flavor!) and soy cheese and spices. Almond butter on sprouted wheat toast, crunchy broccoli soup.

5. Keep a *fresh salad prepared in the fridge*. I always buy pre-washed green salad such as arugula, baby spinach, and romaine lettuce. It's easy to make, I add raisins for sweetness (ditch the bacon bits and croutons though!). To keep your salad fresh in a plastic container, place a folded piece of paper towel on top of the salad, wipe inside cover and replace after each opening.

6. *Use herbs and spices:* Mother Nature has produced incredible flavors, cilantro, basil, oregano, thyme. Any natural spices found at natural food stores.

7. *Drink a few ounces of wheatgrass* per day. Start slow and build gradually. Wheatgrass is available at most health food stores.

8. A fresh smoothie or glass of vegetable juice can more than satisfy a craving.

Since sticking to the above can be challenging and time consuming. *I highly recommend (and take twice daily)* a super-concentrated green drink. The best ones of these are freeze dried living food. The problem with commercial products is that they are not living or alive. It tastes like licking the underside of a lawnmower *but does* miracles as one tablespoon is approximately equivalent to 20 dark green salads!!! They are called super-phytonutrients and include organic oat, Kamut, Barley, Kelp, Aloe Vera and others. Contact me if you want more information. By using these products you give your body what it needs to naturally, safely and easily cleanse itself and build a strong alkaline reserve so no matter **what you eat** you still had your 20 salads and remain alkaline and have access to huge *natural energy*.

3.43 *Fantastic Frequencies : Foods and Organ Systems*

Over the years we have been literally inundated with information on food energy with the measurement of calories. If you're like me the idea of a certain number of calories a day no matter what is completely unrealistic. What if I'm awake longer, worked out, worked extra hard or slept most of the day. What if you are losing weight or building muscle, how do you adjust? A fixed number of calories seems difficult to manage and of little value. I have never measured calories nor believed in them. A great example; many fruits have a very high caloric value, but they are living food and give energy (see chart on page 50). Contrast this to a low calorie cookie, which is dead. If you looked only at calories, you would choose the cookie. Common sense here: which one will give you vibrant energy? The fruit wins always, every time, no exceptions.

A *better, more easily related to and much more manageable way to look at food and energy is a measurement of the food's "life force" energy value measured in hertz, Hz (a frequency). All living things have life force.*

"Some believe the hertz frequency is directly related to how much life force an organism has. For example:

- A *healthy human vibrates at about 62 to 72 MHz,* but *a sick person, depending on how ill he or she is, can dip from 58 MHz* when struck with a minor illness to *as low as 42 MHz* with a major one.

- Degenerative conditions such as *cancer are always detected below 48 MHz.*

- *Illness CANNOT survive in frequencies above 60 MHz."*[20]

According to studies conducted by Dr. Robert Young, and Shelley Redford Young, authors of the brilliant "The pH Miracle"[21] diet book, the website has great alkalizing recipes too! *Foods you include in your diet should ideally have a frequency of at least 70MHz.* Whenever you ingest *any food carrying less than 70 MHz,* you actually use more energy assimilating the food than you get! What this means to you *is that your body keeps craving more food after you eat foods deficient in energy.* Then you crave high calorie "artificial energy" foods such as fried foods, sugary sweets and the drug of all drugs: caffeine! Look at the following chart:

Assorted Food Energies

Food	Frequency (Energy)	Assorted Systems	Frequency (Energy)
Canned Foods	0 MHz	A tumor	30 MHz
Chocolate Cake	1-3 MHz	Liver	55-60 MHz
Fried Chicken	3 MHz	Colon	58-63 MHz
Double cheeseburger	5 MHz	Stomach	58 – 65 MHz
Cooked Vegetables (non-organic)	10 -25 MHz	Top of head	60 – 70 MHz
Cooked Vegetables (Organic)	20 – 25 MHz	Feet	65 MHz
Raw Almonds	40 – 50 MHz	Heart	65 – 70 MHz
Raw Vegetables (non-organic)	70 – 90 MHz	Brain	72 - 78 MHz
Fruits	65 – 75 MHz		
Raw Vegetables (Organic)	70 – 90 MHz		
Live, fresh wheat grass	70 – 90 MHz	Running Computer	90 – 400 MHz
Green Drink	250 -350 MHz	A Rose	320 MHz

So as you can see clearly, living foods should compose the majority of your intake to ensure optimal functioning of all your organ systems. A tumor at 30 MHz is much lower than the healthy range for most organs.

Remember: you can not become ill if you remain above 60MHz!

A recent personal example, I ate at a Chinese food buffet, 4 or 5 plates of the food I used to eat (monosodium glutamate (MSG) -laden food). I was stuffed, but when I got home I was literally famished. This to me proved that eating dead foods not only doesn't nourish us but our body actually says "eat more", since it recognized there is little nutrition and feels it is starving.

3.44 *Great Greens (Includes Yellow and Orange Vegetables)*

Green foods contain almost everything needed for the creation and maintenance of healthy cells. The idea that vegetarians are sickly and weak is simply false. Bottom line, the human digestive track is long like a herbivore (ape), not short like a carnivore (lion). We were meant to eat a predominant diet of fruits and vegetables with some nuts and occasional meat. Here are the reasons why green and yellow vegetables are key to incredible health and energy.

Reason #1: *Phyto-nutrients* are highly active biologically and of great benefit. One large group are called bio-flavanoids, such as allicin in garlic are highly anti-yeast and fungi. High acid diets create fungus and yeasts which feed on sugar and actually increase sweet food cravings!

Reason #2: *Vitamins and Minerals:* Wheat Grass contains more than 100 food elements, including every identified mineral with more iron per volume than spinach! It is 25% protein, higher than meat, dairy, fish, eggs or beans.

Reason #3: *Fiber* comes from plants, vegetables and grasses have a ton of it. Fiber really decreases mycotoxicity (which is the creation of fungi in the human body). Not to mention how important roughage is to cleanse the intestinal tract. Fruit is also a good source of fiber but it is high in sugar which feed fungus' and yeasts and should be minimized, this at least until you become alkaline.

Reason #4: *Vegetables* are a great source of *enzymes.* They are used in all bodily processes. You want to ensure you never run out since they are very hard to make. Enzymes are a part of the overall energy reserve of the body.

Reason #5: Chlorophyll is the blood of plants. Its structure is similar to human hemoglobin which transports oxygen in the bloodstream. Chlorophyll reduces the binding of carcinogens to DNA in the liver, lungs, heart and kidneys.

One of the dominant benefits of *becoming and remaining alkaline* is the phenomenal resilience your body will now exhibit throughout any changes or variable dietary conditions. This will have been built through many months and years of an acid lifestyle building your "alkaline reserves" or "buffer" (Accumulation of beneficial metallic elements in your system). An example of this is my case. I still regularly indulge in the obvious pleasures of popcorn and pop while at the movies. As long as I properly eat a green salad, hydrate and take my green drinks daily, my body seems quite capable of negotiating the random vagaries of a less than perfect, yet real-world diet quite easily with limited after effects. There are always consequences though.

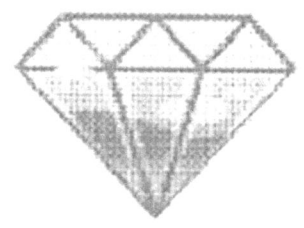

3.5   *5th Diamond :* *Aerobic Energy*

Before I give you my ideas in this area. Let's quickly look at what happens if *you don't exercise.* Some of this may seem self-explanatory, still a good refresher and reminder.

Short/Medium and Long term Impacts of NOT Exercising

Some erroneously believe exercise while growing older destroys the body. *This is false!* If you do not exercise, your system *WILL* fail (disease, discomfort and low quality of life). See the earlier reference on Jack Lalanne.

1. *A sedentary (low movement and exercise) life will shorten your life duration and quality.* Many of my peers (who are tired all the time) don't exercise. The time involved in exercising will *increase* the amount of quality time in your day by allowing you to be less tired and more focused.

2. *Body image issues as well as psychological and emotional lethargy.* I won't lie to you, the *number one reason I exercise is for my mental state!* Having battled my whole life with mood variation issues, I realize the tremendous lift and gift exercising provides me. Sure I enjoy the energy and slim fit look my body has. But whenever I skip a planned and scheduled work out, my mind and emotions are not as sharp, my moods crater. I am a moody person by nature, workouts keep me on the joyful side of moody!

3. *Potential financial costs and losses* associated with lost productivity hours due to fatigue and potential sick time away in surgery, hospital, etc. Just for a moment, how many times last year were you a) on the mend from sickness, b) ill at home missing work or c) just too tired to get through your normal tasks and days?

4. *Dramatically greater risk of muscle and skeletal damage.* Just by living a normal life, walking to the car, sitting, moving, going to the restaurant, shopping, etc. we need our body. If you are not healthy, the odds of damaging your body jump dramatically. We have all heard the story of older (and unhealthy / unfit) people falling/ slipping down icy stairs or sidewalks. They break a hip or clavicle bone. Their recovery can take a full year since their body is weak. If they are healthy, a) they may not have slipped in the first place, b) even if they still slipped/fell the impact would have been much smaller, possibly avoiding a break. I have slipped and fallen many times (I'm a self-avowed klutz!) but rarely broken any bones. I am a bit of a klutz and often slip and fall but rarely get injured due to my body's condition. I did have a painful mountain bike crash 18 months ago and healed extremely well and quickly with minor pain. *When you do get injured, you will heal more quickly and less painfully.*

5. *Reduced Energy levels.* Again, energy is the currency of life. Without it, you can't do/live or experience as much! I don't know about you but as I get older I want to savor every moment as much as possible. Without sounding too arrogant, I can follow the beat / speed of people decades younger than I am due to my high level of energy and health. I can also do more in a day due to not getting tired as easily. How else could I have a full time job and manage 2 companies and write a book. Plus I don't only work. I dine out, travel, see movies, participate in sports. I sleep about 8 hours a night but feel fully refreshed in the morning. If this is not the norm for you, imagine just for a moment that this is not the exception, but fully normal for you too!

6. *Insomnia.* Your body needs to move simply to help all its processes work effectively. If you don't move enough during your waking hours, your body will not be sufficiently tired at bedtime and will sleep poorly. A well-used body has no problems falling asleep and sleep is also more rejuvenating. It's about the contrast. Remember a time when you worked really hard for

a few days on something. Wasn't resting after that much more satisfying.

7. *Reduced Sex Drive.* Now I'm getting personal! Remember how exciting sex was when you were in your 20's? Of course it was new which added to its appeal. But, because you had strong energy, strong hormones and a vitality caused by limited toxins, intercourse was a joy. Also it was often, not once in a blue moon. Sex drive is a personal thing, *however healthy and energetic people have more sex, more often and it is better and less tiring.* Not to even speak of the horrors of many taking a shortcut by not staying healthy and taking erectile enhancers sold by the millions. The risk of a stroke or heart attack is quite a bit higher for someone who is not in good health to have sex increase their heart rate. Also as per point #3, by not being healthy, which makes you happier; you are not in a mood where you want sex. Seriously, *if only for your sex life, exercising is essential! You and your partner will be extremely thankful!*

8. *Increased Muscle Atrophy.* Muscles need to be used. Bones actually need resistance to rebuild stronger. There have been numerous studies with men and women in nursing homes who began resistance training for muscle building. Within 10 weeks they were at 90%+ of the strength most people are at in their 20's, incredible and true!

Bob Delmonteque is chronologically 84 years old, but his body is in the shape of a 30-40 year old, he literally reversed the clock.

"I was 76, that was the best age of my life," he said. " I was so built. My cuts were bulging all over the place. I looked better than any teenager. I could run a 6-minute mile. I won the Senior Olympics in my age bracket. I was just in great shape." Today, "I'm probably in 10 times better shape than anybody my age," Delmonteque added. The doctor of natural medicine still can run a marathon, cycle more than 120 miles a week and bench-press more than 250 pounds."[22]

9. *Increased chance of Cardiovascular disease, high blood pressure, diabetes, cancer and stroke as well as decreased lung capacity.*

3.51 *Health Versus Fitness*

Talk to many people and they will tell you it's better to be fit than to be healthy! Think for yourself, which one is sexier? "I'm really fit!" or "I'm really healthy!" Most would rather be fit than healthy. I myself used to think they were one and the same.

So what's the difference?

Fitness is the physical ability to perform athletic activity.

Health is the state in which all the systems of the body (nervous, muscular, skeletal, circulatory, digestive, lymphatic, hormonal, etc. – are working optimally.

If you want long term energy, health and an absence of aging degradation, the goal is *not to become just fit but healthy.* There are very fit people who ran marathons who were unhealthy and had a heart attack and died. One particular ex US track star died of a heart attack even though she was still regularly running and definitely considered "fit". By being healthy, you will naturally be fitter than the vast majority of people who are unhealthy. *So fitness does not equal health, but health mostly implies fitness.*

To achieve your best possible health and fitness you must train your metabolism. *Many studies have proven that because you exercise consistently over a 12-month (1 year) period, most people become positively addicted to health…for the rest of their life.* In my case I began working out regularly and seriously in 1994. I have never stopped since and don't plan to. I used to get much more muscular and felt I looked ripped. I had many aches and pains, caught colds and needed more sleep than I do now that I am healthy. Now, I work out for health and energy. I fit in the same size pants I did in university. I love shopping for clothes, everything looks slimming! Many people I know go crazy and workout constantly for a year or two then burn out and quit. In health as in all things… slow and steady wins the race. I workout 3-4 times a week (aerobic and weights) plus I walk, play or run with my dog, Riplee twice a day every day.

> **_Health Tip #11_**: **_Fitness_** *is the physical ability to perform athletic activity.*
>
> **_Health is the state in which all the systems of the body (nervous, muscular, skeletal, circulatory, digestive, lymphatic, hormonal, etc. – are working optimally._**

3.52   *Aerobic vs Anaerobic Exercise*

Aerobic means "with oxygen", refers to moderate exercise. The aerobic system gives your body endurance. It contains the circulatory system made up of heart, lungs, blood vessels and aerobic muscles. If you exercise in the "aerobic zone", and eat normally you will *begin to burn fat as your primary fuel! This is what you (and your body) want and need!*

Anaerobic on the flip side means "without oxygen" and refers to exercise that yields power in short surges or bursts. Unfortunately, anaerobic exercise burns a material called glycogen and *causes the body to store fat!* This is definitely *not* what you want!

Your body's *response to a workout*, not the workout itself determines whether or not an exercise is aerobic and anaerobic.

No Pain → All Gain

In my and many trainers' experience, *you are not doing your body any good by creating any pain while exercising!* The objective is to work out lighter but longer and have pleasure. Exercising at 70% of your maximum heart rate rather than 90%, you will be able to workout much longer. The benefit after is you won't feel pain, stressed, destroyed or whipped, you will feel good. Imagine that! Of course you will always see people at the gym on the aerobic machines pushing themselves to the point of exhaustion. I have often wondered, "should I be doing that?" The short answer is *no! Don't do it!*

3.53 *Aerobic Training Advantages: An Impact On the Whole Body!*

A) Your lungs since they work harder become more powerful & more efficient.

B) Increased blood volume means more oxygen supply to the body's tissues.

C) It reduces your risk of dementia and Alzheimer's by 50%, Parkinson's 60%.[23]

D) It reduces your chance of dying from breast cancer (2nd greatest killer of women) by 50%.[24]

E) Creates healthier tissues for better oxygenation leading to less fatigue.[25]

F) It makes the heart more resilient to handle whatever physical and emotional stress occurs.[26]

G) It helps you eat, digest and eliminate waste better through 1500% higher lymph flow with exercise. [27]

H) It helps you sleep better, more deeply with less waking.

I) Enhances physical appearance.

J) Makes you feel better emotionally and mentally.

3.54 *Diets Don't Deliver! Fat in the Body and the Set Point*

Tough news which you already knew (hopefully): *Diets never did, don't and never will work!*

Diets don't work! Why not? *The Set Point.* Nature tends to fight change and wants to preserve its normal levels in all areas! Those who "diet" (reduce caloric, sugar, fat intake drastically) *without exercise* experience the process know as the *"Set Point"*. This is a description of the body's internal mechanism that regulates the amount of fat it keeps in the body. After a few days of decreased caloric intake, the body reacts by decreasing its Basal Metabolic Rate (BMR), this results in more efficient use of the calories.

The automatic biological (self sustaining!) response makes losing weight while dieting progressively more difficult. The body thinks it is starving so it says "Shut all unnecessary processes off until food is available!" If that wasn't scary enough (for dieters of course, you and I know better), the lowering of BMR almost ensures a change physiologically *that makes weight gain easier after the diet!* Once food returns to the body, it says" I missed you, I'm not letting any extra of you slip out again because we may starve!"

"Your body is still working on the basic design outlined millennia ago. It doesn't know that in the industrialized world, food is everywhere. So, when you cut back on your caloric intake, your body automatically thinks there is a famine and will go into starvation mode." [28]

Health Tip #12: Diets alone never have, don't now and will never will work due to the body's Basal Metabolic Rate Adjustment! When you simply lower calories, the body conserves fat!

You *will not lose weight* in a healthy way unless you reset your set point. *The only way to reset your Set Point is exercise!* How? Exercise raises your Basal Metabolic Rate (BMR), the rate your body burns calories. With exercise your body stores less fat than before. Aerobic exercise = more oxygen for energy allowing fat to be burned as fuel and accelerate your metabolic rate to become a veritable fat burning machine.

3.55 *Achieving Aerobic Zone*

Your heart rate during a workout is your key to information telling you whether you are working out aerobically or anaerobically. Thus you should purchase (or find if you have one already) a heart rate monitor to measure your heart rate during exercise.

To calculate your aerobic training range:

i)   Calculate your *Maximum Heart rate : subtract your age from 220.* in my case 220 – 40 = 180. This is your Maximum Heart Rate.

ii) *Calculate your Aerobic Heart rate: 180 – Your Age. So as an example, in my case 180-40 = 140. This number is your Aerobic Training Rate.* Your aerobic rate should be between 60% to 85% of your maximum rate. So in my case: 180 * .7 = 126 beats per minute. As with all new health programs see your doctor and hire an expert: a personal trainer before any major changes to avoid problems.

iii) Lastly to calculate your Warm-up and cool down heart rate= Maximum Rate * 60%, in my case 180 *.6 = 108 beats per minute. Most gyms will give you this information.

3.56   Fat Burning and Muscle Mass

Aerobic exercise is great on its own. However, there is *an enormous incentive* to additionally lift weights to build muscle mass. When you incorporate resistance or weight training you build muscles that burn calories *24 hours a day!* Muscle burns 3 times the calories fat does. Muscle does weigh more than fat in the same space, so your *clothing (waist and posterior) is a better indicator of health than weight is.* Scales indicating body fat percentages are often unreliable in my experience. The traditional caliper method, the ultramodern Hydro Densitometry Weighing Underwater and Bioelectric Impedance methods all give a good measure. I'm not a fan of Body Mass Index calculations as they don't really compensate/distinguish for bone mass or muscle mass. I am considered mildly overweight by this measure!

"In fact, one study published in the Journal of Applied Physiology [6] found that, though weight training doesn't burn as many calories as cardio, it significantly increases average daily metabolic rate - the perfect foundation for losing fat." [29]

As mentioned previously, many also find lifting weights great for the mood and outlook. *Most people do most of their best thinking while resistance (weight) training.* Another thing you can do that builds your brain while building your muscles is listen to motivational speakers on your portable music device. Or you can also listen to music. For women, the often-mentioned rebuttal of "I don't want to get all muscular and bulky" is ridiculous. You would need to work out almost constantly to get that "cut" (muscular). Firmness however will allow you to wear great looking clothes!

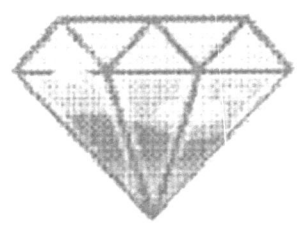

3.6   *5th Diamond*

Ultimate Natural Nourishment

The sad truth for most of us is that we give much more credence and importance to our taste buds than we do to food nutrition and quality, and we pay for it with health problems. Saying *we are unconscious in terms of what we put in our mouths is an understatement.* You don't have to look too far to see people drinking coffee, dairy, soft drinks, alcohol and smoking, eating meat, fried foods, sugar and salty dead food.

Ask most people "why do you eat?", they will answer because they are hungry, because it tastes good and some may even admit they eat because it's there and makes them feel better than their unsatisfying life. My goal for you in this is section to explain the importance of peak nourishment and what happens if we don't apply the principles.

3.61   *Edible Enigma: Why we Eat*

A) **To have energy**: Are you clogging your system or cleansing it? Living, healthy Food gives us the main fuel we need to have the energy to do what we want to do. Good food will allow the machinery to work at its peak so you can do all you need to do and enjoy your life. If your body feels good so does your mood and attitude. Conversely, the wrong foods (for simplicity I include beverages as foods) rob you of energy and leave you sluggish physically and mentally.

B) **To Develop and Grow:**   Our cells are replicated by the thousands of trillions every night when we go to sleep, that's when the body tears down and rebuilds. Think of an analogy of a document being photocopied over and over again at the end of each day: your body's cells do this every night. Your body makes an exact copy of the latest cells it has with the nutrients you absorbed in the day. You want to have the nutrients and minerals available to make great copies that are clearer and sharper than yesterday's, not worse. When people age they are making worse (weaker) copies every day and this leads to degeneration and disease. We must give our body what it needs to regulate and maintain our basic functions. Proper nutrition functions as perfect ink and perfect paper in the machine to complete the analogy. We also need to plan for different stages of our life where our needs can vary.

C) **To Cleanse/Purify:** Don't you want to start each day with a brand new fresh document (photocopy analogy) to draw/paint on? Don't you want to feel refreshed and rejuvenated to leap into your day? You do! Our major *organ systems require cleansing* to work efficiently and powerfully. Quality food helps put a beautiful shine on our exterior shell and largest organ: our skin. Our nails and hair also will regain the sheen they had as children and young adults. Ladies, you can have long flowing hair with many less split ends and the use of a myriad number of chemical hair products.

D) **Prevent and Combat Disease:** As mentioned earlier in 1.91, "the terrain is everything". A healthy terrain via quality nutrition (and hydration) is critical to maintain health and avoid toxifying our body to the point disease takes hold. Food and plants have for thousands of years been used to avoid and cure most ailments from small aches and pains to terminal illnesses. Only over the last 100 years have we turned to modern medicine. Arguably the results are disastrous with more people sick longer than ever.

Unfortunately for us, modern medicine has allowed people to lead mediocre or a below health standard quality of life, much longer!

E) **Socialize and Connect:** Food connects humans together allowing us to love, laugh and share. We unfortunately over-use it to comfort ourselves. As with all things, balance is key so we can feel we have *done our best for our bodies allowing our bodies to do their best for us!*

3.62 *Food Components*

Food is made up of 7 components. These are:

1. **Carbohydrates**: Provide energy via sugars, fiber and starches. The primary fuel for our bodies get broken down into glucose which is the key source of power/energy at the cellular level. Excess carbohydrates become glycogen is then stored in the liver and muscles.

2. **Proteins**, Are made up of animal and plant protein. They are the building blocks of cells. These are known also as the (20) amino acids, 10 of which are considered essential. Amino acids maintain the cells of all the muscles and connective tissues. The liver converts amino acids into a form of carbohydrate when glycogen storage is almost empty.

3. **Fats**, Come in 3 varieties: Saturated, monounsaturated and polyunsaturated. Surprisingly, fats are a very concentrated source of energy (think Eskimos eating seal or whale blubber again). Fats also facilitate the assimilation and absorption of fat-soluble vitamins. Also they insulate the body from toxins and cushion organs from physical trauma. Fats are broken down to Fatty acids, glycerol and cholesterol. *Fatty acids can only be taken in, they can not be manufactured in the body*, Thus their importance.

4. **Vitamins**, Needed to maintain body functions.

5. **Fiber,** don't break down but are useful to scrape the inside of our digestive tract and allow for proper and normal excretion.

6. **Minerals,** As mentioned in section 3.4, Alkalinity, minerals buffer the acid in our body. It is critical to have a large buffer of minerals to maintain the critical acid/alkaline balance. Did you know that when the body's regular buffers are depleted, it (your body) will leach it from your bones! (as it always ensures the body survives no matter what) . Osteoarthritis is this leaching of acid from the bones, on a long term scale.

7. **Water,** We covered the importance of water in section 3.2.

So our goal when we eat, is to eat foods that will facilitate normal bodily functions most. Hopefully with the above information, you will look at your food plate rather differently → to your ultimately your own benefit!

3.63 *Healthy Eating Etiquette*

1. *As children we were told not to drink water while eating.* Of all the myths around food we have discovered/uncovered together so far, this one is very true (i.e. don't drink and eat)! The main reason not to, is that it slows down the digestion process as it dilutes the stomach acid which breaks down food for absorption.

What to do: Drink two glasses of water 30 to a minimum 10 minutes before and after eating meals. The benefits of this are many: a) It will fill you up which will curb your overeating. B) It will allow you the opportunity of breathing correctly (see 3.1 Breathing and Lymphasizing) which helps promote proper digestion.

2. *Food Combination* is probably one of the easiest ways to avoid a number of digestive issues. In order to ensure the best digestion and absorption of nutrients, proper food combination is critical. Ignoring proper food combination will put a strain on our body's ability to digest properly. Problems include A) Uncompleted digestion: This causes food to stop being converted into nutrients which will destroy the body's ability to get assimilate/utilize nutrients. B) Toxins are created which poison the cell and slow the ability of our elimination system to do its job. C) Improper combining can wear down the body and cause graver issues such as acid reflux, ulcers, liver damage, etc. D) Use more energy and feel lethargic. Follow the guidelines below.

The basic principles of food combination: [30]	
Eat a diet that is 70% alkaline, high-water content food and eat only *one* concentrated food (little water content, examples meat, potatoes, chicken or fish.	
1	Protein and carbohydrates should *never* be combined. So meat with vegetables, not potatoes
2	A leafy, green salad can be eaten with *any protein*, carbohydrate or fat.
3	Eat fruits only by themselves and not after any other foods. I.e. eat on an empty stomach. Otherwise they will putrefy (rot) trapped on top of slower-to-digest foods.
4	Fats slow down and hinder the digestion and absorption of protein. If you absolutely must have a fat with a protein, eat a mixed vegetable salad to compensate / offset.
5	Never drink liquids with or immediately following a meal as these will dilute your stomach acids required for proper digestion.
6	Adequate digestion is not possible with the use of condiments such as (but not limited to) vinegar (including salad dressings), alcohol, pop, coffee, iced drinks and tobacco

"Pavlov has conclusively demonstrated that each kind of food provokes a specific, definite type of gastric and intestinal secretion. Because the presence of the three (3) concentrated foods, calls for antagonistic (competing) chemical processes at the same time, it is a physical and chemical impossibility for the digestive glands to function properly as they are subject to definite physiological laws." [31]

Below you will find attached a useful Food combining chart you can post on your fridge.

Food Combination Chart

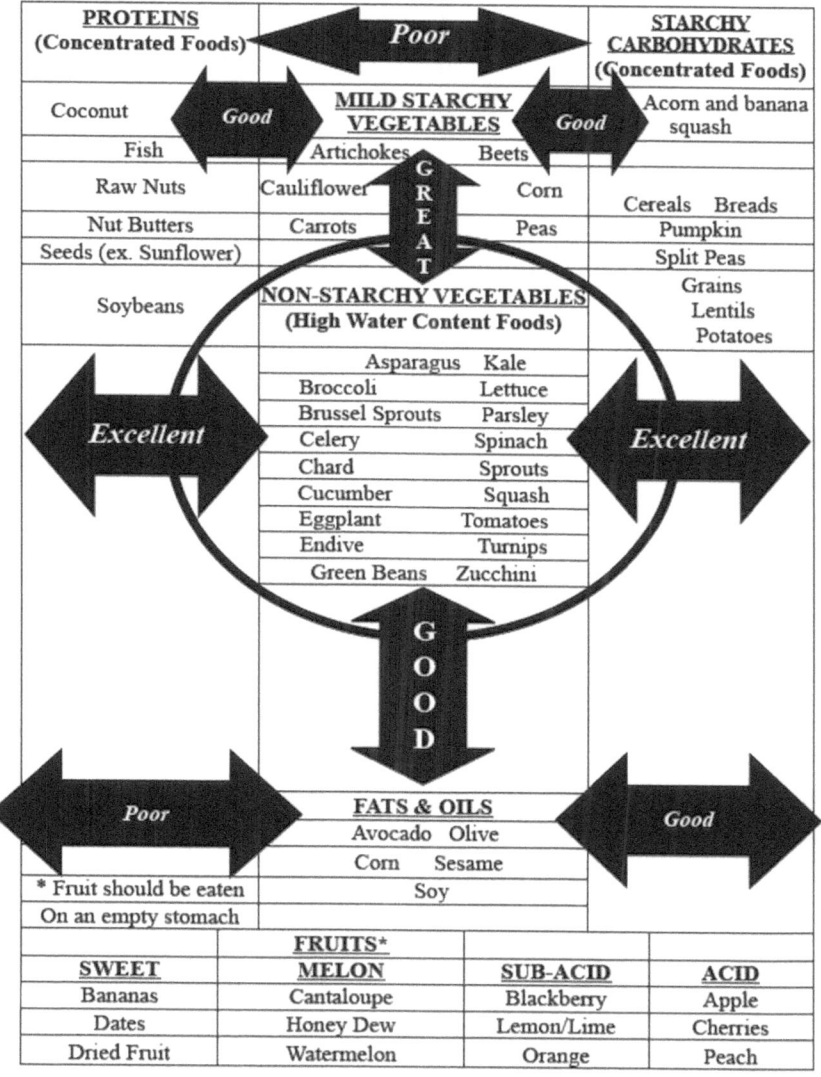

3. *Eat Reasonable Amounts of foods.* Modern serving sizes are completely out of touch with what is required. *Half* the portion served in a typical restaurant dish is what is required. If you cook too much or order too much bring it home and have it for lunch the next day.

For example:	1 cup of pasta	=	size of 1 tennis ball
	½ cup of vegetables	=	the size of a light bulb
	A small baked potato	=	the size of a computer mouse

Reducing caloric intake is said to add years to your life and increase your resistance to illness.

"My doctor told me to stop having intimate dinners for 4. Unless there are 3 other people."
Orson Wells (1915-1985)

4. *Eat in a Relaxed State, Less food BUT more often!* Eliminate distractions including television, cell phones or the internet. Maintain a quiet and serene state. Meals should allow you to appreciate company and the meal. Make sure table is set properly to avoid distractions. Chew food slowly and take smaller bites, this will be necessary if you eliminate water per point number one.

In terms of putting fuel in your car, if you know the tank's capacity is 100 liters, what would happen if you put in 120 liters? The results are obvious! Wasted fuel, money and a dry cleaning bill for your gasoline smelling clothes! As simple as this analogy seems we do this constantly with food, we skip meals then gorge ourselves on too much food. Result: energy drain, lethargy, wasted food, gas, burps etc. Whoever invented 3 meals a day did not live in our modern society with all its time constraints. *A good rule of thumb is to eat small amounts of food every 3 hours.*

Some snacks I use include raw almonds (or soaked in water as per earlier information), dried prunes or figs, whole wheat pita with hummus, celery or carrot sticks. All of these are much more satisfying and healthy than any candy bar or coffee. If you hit an energy wall in mid-afternoon, this is a great indicator you had too much to eat and your body is attempting digestion (one of the most energy intensive processes our bodies complete). Again, drinking 2 glasses of water often cuts the hunger by half easily.

5. <u>*Add supplements to your diet as needed*</u>. See a qualified Naturopath (if you don't have one, get one referred!) on these depending on your specific needs, it's worth it. (See the Supplements Section below).

3.64 *Four Food Group Falsehoods*

The *traditional food recommendations* of most countries should be completely and utterly treated as *outlandish works of fiction!* These recommendations generally fit into "the 4 food groups" or "the food pyramid". Both of these place carbohydrates as the largest food group and then continue to *clog you with dairy and meat servings*. This in no uncertain terms is a *great way to decrease health and increase disease*. The ideal food strategy takes us to back to our roots as grazers on the plains. Remember, 100,000 years is very short in evolutionary terms. Our digestive systems are still the same as they were 100,000 years ago plus or minus minor changes such as dairy issues. We as humans were designed to eat a preponderance of fruits and vegetables (at least 70% live foods), 10% nuts and fish proteins, 10% complex carbohydrates and 10% oils. See "The Biologically Correct Food Pyramid" on the next page.

The Biologically Correct Food Pyramid

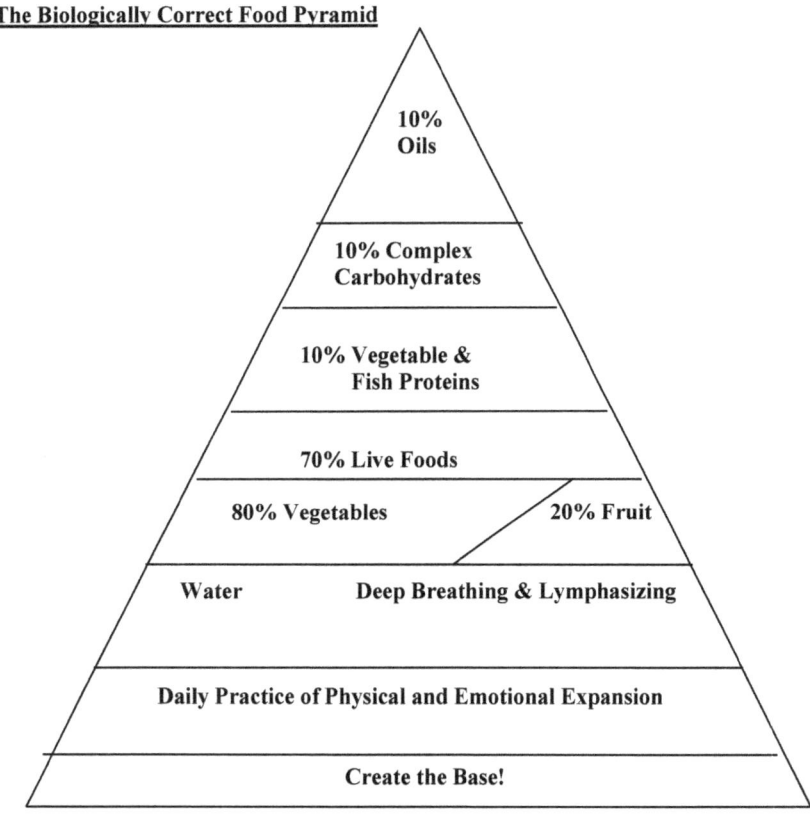

Health Tip #14: *Over 70% of your food intake should be high-water content food (made up of 80% vegetables and 20% fruits).*

3.65   *Sustaining Supplements*

A quick note, *I do not sell supplements and do not own any shares* in supplement companies. In a perfect world, our food would (as it did for countless generations before us) contain all we need in terms of nutrients, minerals and vitamins. A couple of points here: Most people are far from eating a diet remotely close to supplying what they need. No one can have the exact amount of all we need every day. Also, the modern produce we eat gets transported, irradiated, chemically fertilized and coated with all sorts of unknown to nature products. So, better safe than sorry, supplements make a difference. We use supplements to balance out what we need that we don't get from our food. Here is a telling quote:

"Recent evidence has shown that suboptimal levels of vitamins, even well above those causing deficiency syndromes, are associated with increased risk of chronic diseases including cardiovascular disease, cancer and osteoporosis… a large proportion of the general population has less-than-optimal intakes of a number of vitamins, exposing them to increased risk. …it appears prudent for all adults to take vitamin supplements." [32]

Three Levels of Supplements:

First level need to be taken to build a strong base to achieve and/or maintain optimal health. Second level of supplements combat toxins and poisons of our modern lifestyle (did you know you have 13 – 20 lbs of concrete hard fecal matter in your lower intestines?). These help your body naturally cleanse itself as it did before your toxic modern lifestyle. The last group is life period or phase specific.

A) Create the Foundation and Stop the Toxin and Poison Infestation!:

Remember that even *if you do not feel ill, this should not be misconstrued as the absence of disease!* To create a strong base you must stop the poisoning/toxifying and reform and replace the destructive horrible habits that you accumulated. These habits are the wall separating you and perfect, long term, vibrant health. Here are 7 Categories you need to implement.

Essential Oils: As mentioned in section 3.3 products such as Udo's Oil and fish oils (ensure they are from a clean source). I take two high quality salmon oil pills in the morning, these have over 300mg EPA, 600mg DHA. *Cost Approx. $30 per month.*

Digestive Enzymes: If food is not absorbed we don't get any nutrients from our food. Digestive enzymes can help break down food more efficiently. They can help with heartburn, irritable bowel syndrome and other digestive issues. I recommend your nutritionist determine for you based on your challenges. If you do have issues, a natural remedy that helps a stomach ache is *oil of oregano*; it tastes strong but is much more effective and natural than over the counter remedies. I take 1 ounce concentrated cold-pressed Aloe Vera juice. *Do not buy any heat-treated Aloe Vera, it is biologically and nourishment dead!* Aloe helps improve digestion and cleanses the liver. Contact me for my source. *Cost is approximately $40 per month.*

Greens: An alkalizing resource for the body. Wheat and Barley grass as well as Green concentrated Super Phytonutrients. I use and recommend 2 tablespoons (one AM, one PM) of the concentrated super phytonurient (mentioned in Acid Alkalinity section) This product really helps your greens intake no matter your diet, and really helps alkalize your body. Contact me if you want access to these. *Cost is approximately $ 80 per month.*

Multivitamins (Liquid) : Processing and cooking kills nutrients in our food, requiring us to supplement our regimen. One of the *major problems* with traditional multivitamins (along with purity) is that they are absorbed *very poorly* (usually 18%). *Most vitamin companies don't tell* *you this!* So you have expensive pee! I recommend liquid concentrates such as the one I take. These are the best on the market as far as I'm concerned (do your own research!)! These are 88% absorbable. This "anti-aging potion" a high antioxidant fruit beverage with many key cellular regeneration components. This product is unique and an absolute must try for 30 days. Contact me for my source. *Cost is approximately $90 per month.*

Acidophilus: We need good bacteria in our digestive systems, this helps us maintain and achieve a good balance between "good" and "bad" germs in our bodies. I have found I don't need to use this product since I improved my diet.

Anti-Oxidants: Anti-oxidants and vitamins help improve the repair to cell damage caused by free radicals caused by our modern, toxic diets. The above-mentioned antioxidant drink I take is one of the highest available antioxidants on the market. Also in this category are Noni, Acai, Mangosteen and prune juices. Ensure a fresh source (not pasteurized which acidifies and kills the product).

Supplements Based on Your Needs: If you are pregnant or weight training or any other major difference to a "normal" life you may need additional supplements. Additionally, there are an almost unlimited supply of supplements to ease symptoms of specific conditions such as arthritis, etc.

So I do spend almost $250 per month in supplements ($3,000 per year). If this seems high, that is because you don't know, see or feel the way I feel. The amount of quality my life has at 40 is better than I can describe or discuss. I personally am simply not willing to risk my health on always buying the freshest fruits and veggies (which have variable quality levels) even organic. Plus I feel better than I ever have. My perfect health and energy are reasons enough for me. Try it for yourself for 40 days and then make a decision!

> *Health Tip #15: Most multivitamins are not absorbed at more than 18%, expensive urine! Go liquid*

B) Cleansing and Detoxifying Your Body:

Now that you have a strong foundation in place, you are ready and have the pieces in place to a) deal with challenges and b) actually strengthen and get healthier! The solution to ensure lasting and sustainable limitless vitality, energy and health is to take the time to detoxify your body *gently*. The Human body cleanses itself naturally when given the proper nutrients and diet + supplements. The challenge as already discussed at length is the pure acidity of the North American diet and lifestyle. This acid actually encourages micro-organisms such as yeasts (ladies if you get yeast infections you are most definitely acidic!), funguses and spores to grow uncontrolled in your bloodstream! These unwanted "guests" produce *their own wastes (called mycotoxins) adding to your already toxic system!* As if that was not enough, these yeasts cause you to crave sugar snacks such as chocolate, donuts, etc! You can purchase cleansing herbal supplements to achieve a clean system. See your naturopath or trusted natural products source.

C) Milestones to Celebrate Ensure Integration

This part is fun! As with all worthwhile endeavors, you need to celebrate your divorce and destruction of a toxic lifestyle (trust me you'll have the energy to do *this big time!* Set yourself up to win. The reason I push so hard for people to do the 40 Day Plan (see 6.1) is simple. Any sustainable change (including adding or eliminating a habit) take about 4 weeks to become habit, 28 days to be exact.

Part of your odyssey to vital, vibrant and limitless energy is to continuously celebrate and mark key milestones marking your progress. Examples can include your first 10 pounds, your first belt hole adjustment (when you lose inches). Have you always wanted to run a marathon, a 10K, a 5K, etc? Have you wanted to play touch football again, hike a mountain, climb ice falls? Try skydiving, snowboarding and bungee jumping! When you feel as good as I guarantee you will (if you follow my suggestions), *trust me you will!* You *must* celebrate by always improving what you put in your body. It becomes a game with yourself, "What if I cut this?", "What if I add this?". If you want all this to work, a visit to a naturopath and/or reputable health food store will put you in contact with people who live this way *already!* You are now part of the healthy, vibrant, "let's do everything" club. You have left the, "I'm stressed, tired, depressed!" club and may have to rebalance the people you congregate with or risk returning to your toxic lifestyle, *please don't do it!*

3.66 *Negligible Nourishment?*

If we don't eat in a healthy way we continue to literally and figuratively *poison our bodies*. I use poison in a very deliberate manner. Poisoning our bodies via our poor food habits destroys energy, vitality and creates disease. Most people erroneously think *that if they are not ill they are healthy! Remember: Health is not the absence of disease but functioning regularly at your peak.*

You must give your body what it needs in terms of food and supplements, remember that most people spend more on their car than their health. Not eating healthy is as certain a guarantee of ill health as you can take. Most sacrifice medium and long term health for short term pleasure of the taste buds which are so acidified they need really flavorful, chemical filled foods. One month doing what I suggest healthy food tastes will jump out at you and taste unbelievably good.

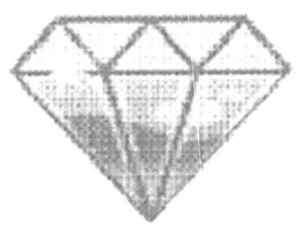

3.7 *Diamond #7 : Alignment & Power*

Have you ever, or do you currently have back pain or any other chronic pain? You're not alone, most people do. Did you ever try standing in one spot for a whole day, do you work as a cashier or security guard, bank teller? Any job that involves standing is a testament to the following: The human body is designed and optimized for motion and movement.

Health Tip #16: The human body was designed and optimized for motion, and a lot of it.

While one may argue we don't gather and hunt on the grasslands anymore, our bodies still need movement and walking/running. In fact *few of us actually ever use the full range of motion that the human body was designed for.*

Maximum health, vitality and energy requires an aligned, flexible, strong body with great muscle tone on the skeleton. When the human body is out of alignment and does not challenge and build the muscles it creates a myriad number of problems with balance, metabolism, visual acuity, fertility and many other key physiological processes. The human body was designed and evolved into a remarkably symmetrical structure. The head is in the middle over the shoulders. The shoulders sit directly over the hips which are firmly placed above the knees. The knees and ankles are perfectly aligned with feet pointed in front.

The Egoscue Method is a way to return the body to its full range of motion.[33] It discusses 7 laws to maximize and optimize the body's structure.

3.71   *7 Egoscue Laws of Structure and Alignment*

1. The Law of Vertical Load: The body's postures must be vertically aligned to leverage the benefits to the body of gravity.

2. The Law of Balance: The body must constantly return to the law of vertical load via muscle memory. Muscles must work in balanced pairs and work equally on both sides of the body.

3. The Law of Compensation: Compensating movements that we are not aware of create problems stealing work from the proper muscles. Functional muscles evenly pass around the stresses and shocks of movements.

4. The Law of Dynamic Tension: The 660 muscles in the body must work to bend the body forward (flexion) and hold it erect (extension muscles) and allow bending backwards. Both must occur at the same time.

5. The Law of Form and Function: Bones do what muscles tell them to do. All motion (skeletal) is begun by muscular activity.

6. The Law of Breath and Oxygen: This law is so key, so essential, the body actually has duplicate and redundant systems to ensure compliance.

7. The Law of Renewal: The body is always in growth and rebirth. All our tissues live. If the body is not renewing it is violating the laws of physical health. The more laws are violated the faster we fall apart, have disease and die.

3.72   *"Core" Strength*

Imagine the core of an apple, the rest of the apple grows out from this core and depends on the stability of the core. Without the core the apple would implode. Your body's core performs the same function, is the foundation for the rest of your body to attach itself and move from. In your body the core is defined as your huge back, chest and abdominal muscles. These are connected to your spine, pelvis and shoulders. They are the base to stabilize your body and coordinate movement.

If your core is weak, this will cause all your external muscles to overstrain and results in many assorted aches and problems. These mostly show up as shoulder and/or back pains. A proper alignment depends on a strong core. Any movement requires strength here, from walking, reaching for food on a high shelf, carrying a baby or throwing a stick. You can do many exercises easily that will strengthen your core. Some you can do at your desk or walking.

__Health Tip #17:__ Strengthen your body's core muscles to minimize random aches and pains and perform better.

3.73 *__Simple Core Exercises__*

- Lie on your stomach arms stretched out in front of you. Raise your left arm and right leg into the air at the same time (ensure chest is slightly off the ground). Hold there for 3 seconds and squeeze your lower back muscles and butt muscles. Repeat with the other arm and leg.

- Try standing balanced on one leg and slowly swing your other leg fore and aft. Avoid twisting and rotation and keep your pelvis vertical. Once mastered, do it with your eyes closed.

- Any simple abdominal exercise will aid core strength. You can hold your ab muscles tight when you shower, walk or drive. Repeat at least 10 times a day.

The only way to grow your overall strength is to build your core.

3.8 Diamond # 8 : Mindset

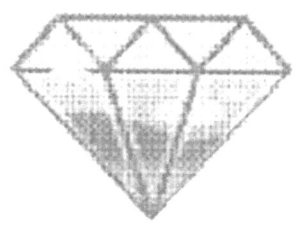

For thousands of years, witch, shaman and/or medical doctors did not have access to modern medical technologies, surgical instrumentation or modern chemical mixtures to "heal" sick people. They focused on the body's natural, internal war machine to raise its resistance, fight disease and maintain/recreate health. In many ways those primitive methods were superior to today's results. These ancient healers realized and maximized the power of a directed and present mind. Channeled and focused in a positive direction, our mind, thoughts and emotions can be powerful tools in our quest to become or remain vibrant and healthy. As mentioned much earlier fear is a toxic emotion which puts our body in a state of high alert. This is useful if a bear is chasing us as we physically use the adrenaline. However when the fear is imagined these hormones create stress and break down our *body just as much as a poor diet!* We all know people who eat constantly and stay fit and others who barely touch food and gain weight. Our mindset is powerful in the search for complete, vibrant and radiant health._

> ### Health Tip #18: *Worry, stress and fear about your health are AS toxic as a poor lifestyle.*

If we don't do the psychological work around dealing positively with our coping skills and social support we remain at risk to all forms of mental illness which quickly degenerate into physical illness. The mind and our imagination are a part of the body and can create fear in our body as much as a real fear would. When our body is stressed (as if often is at the traditional holiday period) our internal balance is upset and our resistance is lowered. The more vulnerable we are the greater at risk we are.

"A bodily disease which we look upon as whole and entire within itself may, after all, be but a symptom of some ailment in the spiritual part."

Nathaniel Hawthorne

We have the choice of how we react to any situation, *it is the meaning we assign (our interpretation) to what happens that is important NOT the event itself.* Our mind and behaviors, our environment, and our genetic makeup are the common contributors to disease. The way we react to the daily trials and tribulations (not to mention stressful major life events) of our life determine the difference in between "coming down with" an infection, cold or remaining healthy. Since most of the microbes that afflict us are already residing in our bodies, they are only a part of the cause of illness if combined with other risk factors that create a proper "terrain" for illness to "grow". A risk factor may be a toxic diet, smoking, alcoholism or a permanently negative ("life is hopeless and out of my control") life view. We are much more careful about what we watch on TV than the thoughts we let into our minds.

3.81   The Power and Unique Intelligence of Your Heart

Most of us know the brain controls most autonomic bodily functions (breathing, digestion, etc.). Did you know however that the heart has its own brain! Yes, modern research has proven that the human heart communicates with the brain and the body *as a separate entity.*

- *The heart actually sends more messages to the brain than the brain sends to the heart!*

- The heart communicates in 4 ways: 1) neurologically (electrically), 2) biophysically through the pulse (a form of pressure wave), 3) biochemically through hormones (includes Oxytocin, the love hormone!) and 4) an energetic communication (electromagnetic).

- Few people are aware that the heart has its own separate nervous system.

- *The heart has its own electrical field*, you can see the difference in heart rate variability between the attitudes of Appreciation (coherent and predictable field) and Frustration (incoherent, jagged unbalanced field). For example, did you know that only 5 minutes of anger takes 6 hours of calm to return your heart back to its coherent electrical field pattern. Getting and staying angry actually stresses your body dramatically.

Health Tip #19: *Don't get angry! Just 5 minutes of anger takes 6 hours of calm to return your heartbeat's electrical field back to normal. Stress ACTUALLY DOES KILL!*

When you are feeling caught up in a negative or disempowering pattern of emotions, one of the quickest and most powerful remedies is to balance your nervous system through breathing through your heart. Here is how to do this:

1. Shift your focus to the area around your heart

2. Imagine and feel your breath coming in through your heart and out through your solar plexus.

3. Activate positive feelings and emotions by embodying them while breathing through your heart. [34]

"When you use your heart intelligence to shift perceptions and direct the flow of your emotions, you have the ability to generate and magnetize your own fulfillment." [35]

Doc Childre & Howard Martin

4.0 The 4 Destroyers / Dinosores Of Health : Poisons/ Toxins That Kill You

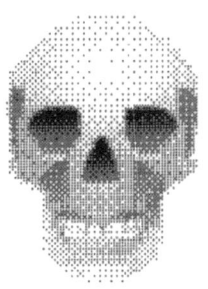

The 4 Dinosores (Destroyers) of Health

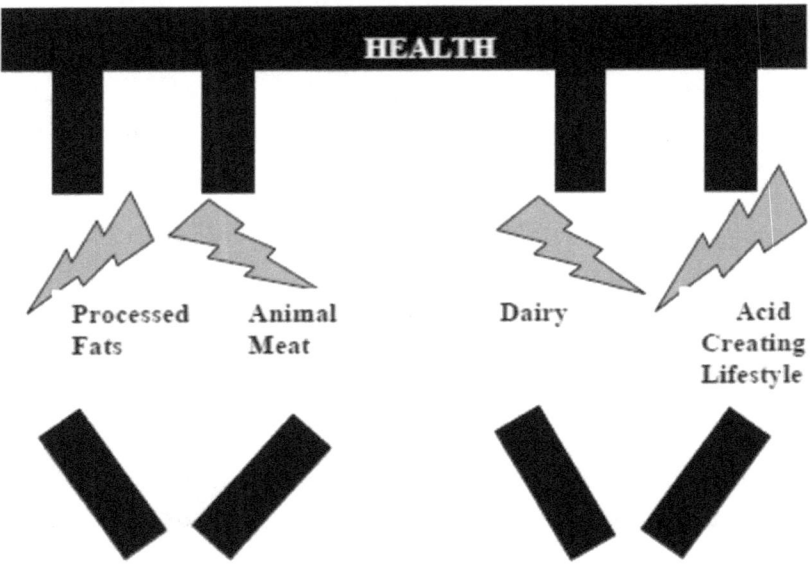

So, if your full, optimal vibrant health is likened to a sturdy wooden table. The following 4 Destroyers of Health are like termites, rot, or axes which cut your health, energy and lifespan dramatically. They are toxins that poison you and kill you more quickly than any other. In business it is often said to focus on the 20% of actions that create 80% of the results. Following are the 20% of things that if you eliminate will give you 80% of improvements in your energy, vitality and health. Handle these, and you will literally be reborn. Similar to everything I have proposed in this book, do as I did, don't take my word for it, try it in your own body and see! Again, always under the supervision of a health professional.

4.1 *Dinosore 1 :*
Toxin 1: Processed Fats

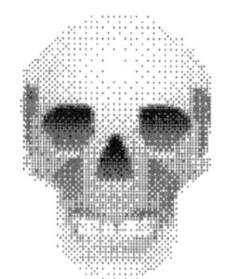

Butter, margarine, cheese, French fries, chips, cookies etc, etc. Makes the mouth water doesn't it? So what's so bad about these "harmless" little treats? I can see your face right now, Cheese, cookies??!? What's next?! Wait. Processed Fats are the main flavor creators in the above foods as well as others. These fats can be made via chemical cooking to taste like virtually anything. Think in the lines of: they could make cardboard really flavorful, tasty and addictive. As mentioned earlier; the lion's share of fats we eat are saturated, polyunsaturated, monounsaturated and trans fatty acids. *North Americans generally obtain about 35% to 40% of their total calories from fat.* These fats *raise blood cholesterol.* Unless you just arrived from a small lost island in the south pacific, you know *blood cholesterol is the major risk factor* for coronary heart disease which leads to heart attacks and stroke.

Processed or Trans Fatty Acids:

Man-made or processed fats, manufactured from liquid oil. When hydrogen is added under pressure to liquid vegetable oil the result is a *stiff, non-pliable fat.* This rigid and stiff fat is very similar to the fat found in a can of Crisco. Trans fats equal hydrogenated fats.

4.11 *Terrible Trans Fats*

In study after study, it has been proven that *trans fatty acids (hydrogenated fats) raise total blood cholesterol and LDL (so-called "bad") cholesterol and lower HDL ("good") cholesterol* when used instead of naturally occurring fatty acids or natural oils. These differences increase the risk of heart disease. According to the comprehensive Nurses'

Health Study [36], the largest investigation of women and chronic disease; *Trans fats double the risk of heart disease in women.* A recent 10-year study showed *similar results with men* eating the most trans fats having twice the risk of hear attack. Other trans-fat bugaboos include poor circulation, poor elimination, excess mucus formation and toxicity in the body. If that wasn't enough, *food manufacturers put chemicals that guarantee you will never be satiated eating their product so you eat more and more,* you get little to no nutritional value. These chemicals are not only toxic, but they are highly addictive.

If you don't think trans-fats are bad, do yourself a favor and rent the 2004 documentary, "Supersize Me". [37] This excellent documentary dramatically shows the dangers of a fast food lifestyle. The main character goes on a "fast food only" diet for a month, *the drastic negative changes in his cholesterol, energy, weight, mood and sex drive were unbelievable.* Also, he was craving fast food constantly and getting massive headaches. His doctors warned him to stop, as he was literally dying from the Trans fat and sugar, within 3 weeks! Only an independent person could have ever subjected themselves to such a frightening test.

The more you eat, the more work you create for your body with no nutrients to fuel it. *As a contrast, try eating more than 2 bananas, you can, but it will be hard as there are natural compounds that tell your brain: "I'm full, stop eating!"* I can't remember any tub of popcorn, ice cream or chips telling me I was full!

> ___Health Tip #20___: **Consuming trans fats in butter, margarine, cheese, fries, cookies, etc. double (+100%) the risk of heart disease in men and women.**

Remember: Not all Fats are bad!

As covered in section 3.3, Essential Oils, *we need* "good" unsaturated fats including Omega 3 and 6 fatty acids that help reduce the risk of heart disease and cancer. *Easy rule here, if it's been modified at a high temperature➔ it's not good for you.* Good fats actually help build cellular walls.

The American Heart Association's Nutrition committee strongly advises that healthy Americans *over age 2* (in other words, everyone!) limit their intake of saturated fat and Trans fat to less than 10% of total calories. This is three (3) to four (4) times less than the typical North American eats. The FDA also has forced manufacturers to list these on all products since January 1st, 2006.

Most of us are literally digging our graves with our teeth and killing ourselves with our forks!

4.12   *Daily Trans Decrease*

1. Replace butter with olive oil and garlic. Try almond butter rather than peanut butter.

2. Eliminate or greatly reduce cookies, pastry and crackers.

3. Limit intake of snack foods and chips. Replace with chewy and crunchy dried fruits (raisins, figs and prunes) and almonds.

4. Avoid deep fat fried foods and fried foods in restaurants, go baked or broiled. If you must eat, have a huge salad to counteract. Add flax seed oils to your meals.

5. Eliminate packaged, convenient foods. Create guacamole with avocados, lemons and garlic, a delicious and healthy dip!

4.13   Torrid Temperatures Turn Fat Toxic

Fats that are destroyed at over 45 degrees Celsius (118 degrees Fahrenheit) are called *Processed Fats*. They are at this point *completely unusable and toxic to the human body.* This increases acid formation and disease producing conditions in your body. Examples include whole milk, meats, butter, margarine, cheese, etc. These cause poor circulation (which causes high blood pressure), poor elimination (toxicity remains in the body too long), excess congestion (due to mucus creation). Also the body is not able to perform its tasks and functions that good fats provide.

4.14   *Processed Fat Contents vs Natural Fat Contents*

Processed Vs Natural Fat Percentages

% OF CALORIES AS PROCESSED FAT		% OF CALORIES AS NATURAL FAT	
MEAT		**VEGETABLES**	
Turkey, Dark meat with skin	**47%**	Potato	**1%**
Chicken, dark meat with skin, roasted	**56%**	Artichoke	**3%**
Hot Dog	**80%**	Green bean	**6%**
Bologna	**81%**	Asparagus	**6%**
Bacon (lean)	**81%**	Cauliflower	**7%**
Sirloin steak, hipbone, lean with fat	**83%**	Cabbage	**7%**
		Mushroom	**8%**
FISH		Lettuce	**12%**
Salmon, sockeye red	**49%**		
Caviar, Sturgeon	**52%**		
Black Sea Bass	**53%**		
Tuna, chunk, oil-packed	**63%**		
DAIRY PRODUCTS		**NUTS AND SEEDS**	
Low fat milk (2%)	**31%**	Sunflower seeds (raw)	**64%**
Cottage Cheese	**35%**	Pumpkin seeds (raw)	**68%**
Regular Ice Cream	**48%**	Hazel or Brazil nuts	**70%**
Whole Milk	**49%**	Raw Almonds	**76%**
Eggs Whole	**65%**		
Swiss cheese	**66%**		
Cheddar Cheese	**71%**		
Cream Cheese	**90%**		
Butter	**100%**		

The differences are completely staggering! [38]

4.15   *Figuring Fat Percentage*

To estimate the percentage of calories from fat you are consuming, multiply the grams of fat by 9 (the # of grams of fat in a calorie) and divide by number of calories.

Example: Local yogurt, 10 grams of fat (10) in a serving X 9 = 90 and divide by total number of calories (210).

Formula: (# of grams of fat X 9) / # of calories = % calories of fat

For optimal health, daily fat intake should always be less than 25%

4.2   *Dinosore 2 : Toxin 2 :*
Animal Flesh/Meat

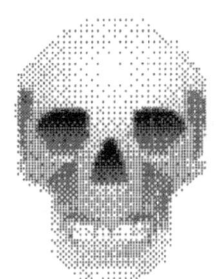

Don't get me wrong, I am *not* one of those
lifelong vegans, whom I used to ridicule (my
apologies, I was young and ignorant!), far from
it. I used to eat meat almost 3 times a day, from
bacon and eggs or toasted waffles in the morning, to burger at lunch
to beef/pork or chicken at night. I have never liked fish or seafood. I
love beef steak, really, it is my *favorite meal possible, bar none.* I love
it cooked in a primal fashion on the barbeque with steak sauce and/
or Béarnaise or peppercorn sauce. I have often said to anyone (who
would listen!), (and I still believe,) if I was on death row and had but
one final meal, steak and fries would be that final meal. I'm saying this
so you can clearly see I'm not a person who always hated meat or grew
up vegan, *far from it.* I still eat meat, but have reduced it dramatically
(85% +). You will soon understand the reasons why I took this, for me
at least, (and maybe for you as well) quite drastic step.

Meat is a staple of the North American diet, *so much so,* most people
may believe a life without steak, cheeseburgers, chicken wings and
ribs is not a life. The opposite is actually true, meat is destroying and
shortening people's lives.

"My favorite animal is steak!"

Fran Lebowitz (1950 -)

Again, at the risk of repeating myself, *if you want the same results as
everyone else, keep eating what they do!* The fact is, traditional eating is
killing people in massive proportions so we need to change (if we chose
a quality life). Simply look at the rates of heart disease, cancer, obesity,
diabetes and more around in your circle of family and friends, this is
usually a more powerful wake up call than nebulous distant statistics
on the late night news. Look around your life, how many people are

suffering from obesity, heart disease, cancer, stroke or diabetes among other ailments. *Shifting to a plant-based diet is the fastest way to health and almost as importantly really the only sustainable option.*

"Nothing will benefit human health and increase the chance of survival of life on earth as much as the evolution to a vegetarian diet."
Albert Einstein

In the book "The Food Revolution: How Your Diet Can Help Save Your Life and Our World"[39], John Robbins presents the following alarming statistics on a meat-based diet.

Heart Disease:

- Heart Disease deaths for vegetarians compared to non-vegetarians: Half. (50% Less!)

- Blood cholesterol drop of 14%

- Drop in heart disease for every 1% decrease in blood cholesterol: 3-4%.

- Incidence of very high blood pressure in meat eaters compared to vegetarians: *1300% higher!*

Cancer:

- There is a *20% to 60% reduction* in lung cancer risk for people who *frequently eat green, orange and yellow vegetables.*

- Most common cancer for American men: prostate cancer. Risk of prostate cancer for men whose intake of cruciferous vegetables (broccoli, Brussels' sprouts, cabbage, cauliflower, collards, kale, mustard green and turnips) is high: *41% reduction*

- Risk of colon cancer for women who eat red meat daily compared to those who eat it less than once a month: *250% greater.*

4.21 Immense Impact and Implications

Startling Implications for Diet, Weight Loss and Long-Term Health [40]

Scarier than any horror movie since this is *not fiction!*:

- American society spends more per capita on health in the world yet *67% of Americans are overweight.* In Canada 44.8% of Canadians are overweight.[41]

- Over 15 million Americans have diabetes, the heart disease level has not decreased one percentage point in the last 30 years. This is alarming since we have so much modern equipment and chemistry and knowledge. This means the situation is getting worse not better despite billions of dollars and human capital hours invested.

- Half of all Americans take a prescription drug every week.

- 100+ Million Americans have high cholesterol

- Greater than 33% of young Americans and 32% of Canadian teens[42] are overweight or at risk of becoming overweight.

The majority of the above challenges come down to one source: Nutrition! Cancer, heart disease, diabetes, and many other diseases that plague modern society, *can in fact be prevented as well as treated by a whole foods, plant-based diet.*

Health Tip #21: *Cancer, heart disease, diabetes, and many other diseases that plague modern society, can in fact be* prevented *as well as* treated *by a whole foods, plant-based diet.*

The authors benefitted from a 27 year grant from the National Institute for Health (NIH), the American Cancer Society, and the American Institute for Cancer Research (the largest and most comprehensive health and nutrition study ever conducted) found the following regarding (non-plant) protein:

- Low-protein diets prevented the initiation of cancer by aflatoxin, a toxin found in peanuts and corn. *Did you know aflatoxin is considered in the general medical community as one of the most potent carcinogens ever discovered?*

- Once cancer is initiated, *low animal protein diets dramatically blocked subsequent cancer growth.* I have heard of living examples of people with huge cancerous tumors who were "diagnosed" as terminal by traditional medicine. *Once these persons turned to a high living food diet within weeks the tumors completely disappeared as did all symptoms!* Do not ever leave a diagnosis to *only one* medical professional. *You are the true expert on your body, don't give that power away! All medical diagnoses should be considered opinions and not facts.* Virtually every disease known to man can be treated via wholesale changes in lifestyle and minor natural plant substrates. Do your own homework and try it with your own body and see the spectacular results.

- *Cancer was consistently promoted by casein, which makes up 87% of cow's milk.*

- Even at the highest levels of intake, "safe" proteins from plants *did not* promote cancer.

The body needs protein and builds most of the proteins it needs from amino acids. *"Low-quality" plant protein,* which allows for slow but steady synthesis (building) of new proteins, *is the healthiest type of protein.*

My opinion here, is that the findings point to the same conclusion: *people who consume the most animal-based food get the most chronic diseases, and that even small amounts of animal-based foods cause adverse effects.*

__Health Tip #22__: People who consume the most animal-based food get the most chronic diseases, and that even small amounts of animal-based foods cause adverse effects.

4.22   *Obesity: Globally Gross Girth*

According to the World Health Organization, the number of obese adults *grew 50%* from 1995 to 2000! Obesity is defined by the Center for Disease Control (CDC) as individuals with a Body Mass Index of 30 or above. A BMI of 25 to 29.9 alerts to being overweight. You can calculate your own BMI at the CDC website:

http://www.cdc.gov/nccdphp/dnpa/healthyweight/assessing/bmi/adult_BMI/english_bmi_calculator/bmi_calculator.htm

Obesity has already overtaken smoking as the leading cause of death in the United States according to the CDC. Even more alarmingly, developing countries are now shifting their diets to a more high-fat diet recreating the same problems we see here. More than 115 million people in developing countries have obesity-related problems.[43]

The most staggering statistics belong to children in industrialized nations. About 20% of American children are clinically obese. This dramatically increases Type II Diabetes (the type that occurs when we are severely overweight). Find a way to limit television and video games for your kids and encourage outdoor sports or other vigorous activities. My opinion is that it is one thing for adults to choose an unhealthy lifestyle as they are free to do what they want. When it comes to overweight children, I become seriously angry, since the children never had a chance, they were never shown a healthy childhood. In my view, if your kids are overweight, you are stealing much of the joy and energy of childhood, saddling them with long-term self-esteem and health issues. *So if you don't get healthy for yourself, do it for your kids!*

Weight Loss Ideas:

- Take the stairs rather than the elevator
- Walk or bike to places instead of driving
- Get a dog (Rain, snow or shine you can get a couple of walks and relaxation every day!)

- If you have to drive, park further away so you can get some exercise.

- Instead of TV and Movies, try kickboxing and dancing!

4.23   *Protein Propaganda!*

Fact or Fiction Regarding Animal protein

A) "I need to eat animal protein to have a complete and balanced diet." → FICTION

If you are like most people, if someone mentions the word "protein", immediately your mind thinks meat! Animal protein *does not* have to be a part of your diet to obtain protein. Vegetarians have always and continue to obtain *healthier and more* protein from a plant-rich diet! Even the USDA admits that "protein needs can easily be met by eating a variety of plant-based foods. Combining different protein sources in the same meal *is not necessary or even recommended*. Dark Green vegetables (such as broccoli, kale, spinach, etc.) are rich sources of protein (remember Popeye eating spinach to get super-strong to save Olive Oil (who also had a healthy name!)?). For example, broccoli is 51% protein! A diet of these vegetables will *more than adequately* meet all your protein needs.

Have you noticed young girls of 9 and 10 years old beginning to show signs of puberty? You're not hallucinating, they are! This is happening 3 to 5 years earlier than it (normally) used to. Why? There are a multitude of hormones fed to crops then to animals we eat (and through the milk kids drink!). So much so, American and Canadian beef are banned in Europe due to the hormones! [44]If it isn't not good enough for Europe why is it good enough for you and I?

"The European Economic Community banned hormone-raised meat because of questions on the dangers of meat that has been treated with synthetic sex hormones. European consumers pressured the EEC to take this action to protect their health warned of the carcinogenic risks of estrogenic additives which can cause imbalances and increases in natural hormone levels." [45]

Also, we know antibiotics are bad for humans, but our meat is filled with antibiotics to ensure they grow quickly without illness and less exercise.

"Ranchers and farmers have been feeding antibiotics to the animals we eat since they discovered decades ago that small doses of antibiotics administered daily would make most animals gain as much as 3 percent more weight than they otherwise would. In an industry where profits are measured in pennies per animal, such weight gain was revolutionary." [46]

B) *"Protein should be 20% to 30% of my daily diet." → FICTION*

Different studies (NRC, USDA and WHO) advise between <u>4% to 8% protein</u> (and not specifically animal protein!).

> ***Health Tip #23:** A Healthy diet should contain between 4% to 8% protein only (plant protein being the dominant percentage).*

C) *"I need to eat Protein to have Energy!" → FICTION*

The human body burns materials in this order: 1) sugar first, 2) carbohydrates second, 3) protein 3rd. Additionally, too much protein creates nitrogen which is a primary cause of fatigue.

D) *"Yes, but I'm an athlete/workout fanatic! I can't have the strength and endurance to perform while eating as a vegetarian!" → FICTION*

Many world-class athletes would very strongly disagree including 7 time Ironman winner Dave Scott, tennis God Martina Navritilova, weight lifter Bill Pearl, Heisman Trophy winner Desmond Howard and legendary Energizer Bunny motivational speaker Anthony Robbins.

E) *"Some of the Most Respected and Powerful Animals Are Meat-eaters!" → FICTION*

Look at nature, one of the most powerful animals pound per pound in nature is the gorilla, generally regarded to be 5 to 10 times stronger than a human, it eats leaves and fruits! The gorilla, being a primate is the closest anatomically to a human of all animals. Those who site animals such as big cats forget to mention that lions for example have small intestines that are 3 times their body lengths versus 6 times for a human. What this means is that the human digestive process is 12-18 hours long (versus 4 hours for Lions and other big cats). This causes meat to decay and form free radicals which destroy cells and cause degenerative diseases, premature aging and cancer.[47] Do you have 22 hours to lounge around every day to digest? Meat protein is the most energy intensive of all digestive processes as it requires many different types of enzymes. Eat a huge protein meal and then *forget about being productive!* Even black bears derive only a minute amount of their food from animal proteins (even then they eat insects!).

F) *"Protein Needs are the Greatest as an Infant"* → *FACT*

Despite this, less than 2% of mother's milk is protein. As an adult, what is the food group closest in protein percentage to 2%? The answer is *fruit!* As the human body grows it becomes more efficient and actually learns to recycle protein itself.___

4.24   Environmental Excesses!

An animal-based diet threatens our environmental resources. Without even mentioning the pollution farm animals create on water systems. Without mentioning that 1 quarter pound hamburger requires clearing 6 square meters of rainforest, the destruction of 65 kilograms of living matter including 20 to 30 plant species and dozens of birds, insects and reptiles. [48]

Every pound of beef you avoid equals 12,000 to 20,000 liters of water. Huge amounts of Carbon Dioxide are produced. Wrap your head around this: *Eating 1/4 pound (100 grams) of hamburger does the same damage as driving your car for more than 5 days!* [49]Additionally, raising animals for meat is one of the largest contributors of methane gas pollution on the planet. As the BRICK countries (Brazil, Russia, India, China and South Korea) espouse the lifestyle of the western countries this huge impact (destruction) on the planet will actually become one of the greatest challenges to our planet.

> ___Health Tip #24:___ *Eating one 1/4 pound (100 grams) of hamburger does the same environmental damage as driving your car for more than 5 days! Help the planet, reduce!*

4.25   Choking on Chicken Challenges

A disclaimer here, I still eat chicken occasionally, but limit it to a few times a week maximum.

It has been a generally accepted fact that chicken is safer/healthier than beef. This is *incorrect*. Due to many factors, eating chicken is in many ways worse than consuming beef. Along with the hormone and antibiotic issues mentioned earlier for beef, a myriad of other challenges in growing and processing chicken almost ensure this meat is ripe for corruption/poisonings of many types.

You don't need to be an animal owner or lover to be horrified by the following. Did you know chickens are jammed into miniscule cages 4 per cage so they can't flap their wings or stand? Their beaks are ripped off without anesthetic to stop them from injuring each other in these horrible conditions. Did you also know they are fed growth hormones and artificial lighting which cause them to *outgrow their own bones* resulting in painful fractured and broken bones for the animal.

Once they are grown they are exposed to many levels and types of contamination on their way to their fearful and inhumane deaths. They are dumped into boiling tanks which finally puts them out of their misery. An important detail here. The chickens when they land in the scalding tanks literally soil themselves and the huge amount of fear in them is locked into their meats. You don't have to be spiritual to realize eating a terrified animal's fear brings some of the fear into you. The chickens are then de-feathered and submerged in a chilled holding tank often called "fecal soup". This soup is ripe with the wastes the animals created upon death and is a cesspool for bacteria. Here's the kicker that did it for me: *The Uric acid (from the urine the animal created upon scalding) is what gives chicken (and beef) its texture and taste.* The chewy consistency and texture of beef and chicken are byproducts of the putrefactive germs that tenderize the meat. These colon germs, flood the animal once it is killed and soften the tissues to be appealing to the pallet of the meat consumer.

Here is a quote from a former USDA microbiologist Mr. Gerald Kuester.

"With the advent of modern slaughter technologies there are about 50 points during processing where cross-contamination can occur. At the end of the line, the *birds are no cleaner than if they had been dipped in a toilet.*" [50]

__Health Tip #25__ : Avoid Chicken! It is one of the worst meats. If you must eat it, ensure a kosher, Hallal, free range or organic source.

Had enough? Here's a little more if you're still in doubt. Agriculture Department studies have shown that 99% of broiler (chicken) carcasses have detectable levels of E. coli, 30% have Salmonella and over 70% campylobacter (a cause of food poisoning and gastroenteritis, diarrhea, fever, etc.). [51]

4.26   Meat Mastery and Management

Hopefully the above information (though shocking and hair-raising) has gotten you to re-balance your ideas around meat and it's inverse relationship to health. If you are like me, you can see yourself drastically limiting chicken and other meat intake. Total abstinence is often impractical and feels like it limits your pleasure to have/share many foods.

If you must eat meat take the following precautions.

A) Eat and limit your animal flesh intake *to one meal a day,* maximum. It would be better at lunch as it will give you longer to assimilate it!

B) Properly combine your food as per Section 3.63 (no meat with carbs!). Also *eat your meat with a large portion of water-rich foods. (NO, fries don't count!)* Ensure you have a *large* salad and or steamed vegetables (I usually ask them to replace potatoes with more vegetables), sides that clean, not clog you. Try to eat a cleansing diet for the rest of the day.

Health Tip #26: _If you must eat animal flesh, eat it at lunch, maximum once a day and with a huge salad or steamed veggies (avoid carbohydrates)!_

C) **Choose meats that are: 1) Free range, 2) Kosher or Halal, 3) Antibiotic-free, Organic.** As mentioned earlier, these meats will barely have any taste (due to lack of Uric acid and will require more seasoning and flavorings). These meats also avoid the animal terror associated with all other methods.

D) **Have seafood:** It's a great source of protein, essential fats, and nutrition as long as you can guarantee a natural and clean source. If unclean, large amounts of lead and arsenic await you.

E) **Stay Alkaline:** Once your body is alkaline, many "salty" cravings, especially meat will disappear. See section 3.4 on Alkalinity.

F) **Avoid Processed "Meats":** These are not meat! These include hot dogs, pepperoni any and all deli meats. The amount of bad meat that goes into these products combined with the potential for infection make these an extremely poor choice for eating at any time. The two reasons processed meats are so bad are 1) the huge amount of saturated fat in the "meats" which concentrate the toxins of the food the animal eats and 2) Sodium Nitrate is a cancer promoting additive.

"…the USDA actually tried to ban this additive (Sodium Nitrate) in the 1970's but was vetoed by food manufacturers who complained they had no alternative for preserving packaged meat products. [52]

Processed meats are proven to increase the risks of colorectal cancer dramatically. Summer barbecue season, limit hot dogs to 2 a month. .

4.3   *Dinosore 3: Toxin 3: Dairy Foods and Liquids*

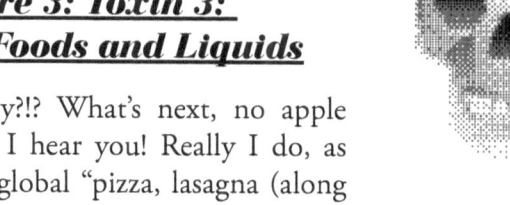

Dairy?!? Dairy?!? What's next, no apple pie or baseball?!? I hear you! Really I do, as a founder of the global "pizza, lasagna (along with Garfield) and nachos" fan club, this one was even tougher than meat for me! However, drastically reducing dairy products (for many including myself, at least) has been the one that gave me the greatest positive impact. I have struggled with gassiness, allergies, phlegm and asthma for most of my life. Allergies to pollen, cut grass, cats, dogs, dust etc. plagued me for my whole life. Since I gave up (90%) dairy (includes milk, cheese, yogurt), these symptoms have mostly (90%) disappeared and a new limitless energy has replaced it. *Again, don't listen to me, try it for yourself and trust your body!* Go 40 days without dairy (definitely, no less than 10 days) and then become a believer as I did.

4.31   Dairy Destruction Demons: How Dairy Disintegrates You

A) **Cancer:** All mammals create milk. Milk is a great medium for transportation of chemicals including the hormone, insulin-like growth factor 1 (IGF-1). Milk consumption dramatically increases the circulating levels of IGF-1. Increased levels of this hormone are strongly related to prostate cancer, colorectal cancer, breast cancer (premenstrual) as well as lung cancer. In 9 separate studies, the greatest (and most consistent) dietary factor linked with prostate cancer was a high consumption of milk and/or dairy.

B) **Mucus Production:** Both milk and dairy products generally tend to contribute to the production *of excessive mucus in the sinus, lungs and intestines.* This extra mucus in the intestines becomes almost cement-like in density as well as impermeable to nutrients *(this means you eat and are starving to death as not enough nutrients are absorbed!)*. This in turn leads to weak absorption, which creates a condition of chronic fatigue. Drinking milk also creates excessive nasal dripping and throat phlegm. I have noticed a dramatic reduction in throat and nasal moisture since I greatly reduced the intake of dairy products. Vegans eliminate milk for the same reasons.

C) **Allergies:** Not too many people properly metabolize cow's milk protein. Up to 10% of asthma cases could be connected to food allergies. Food allergy is the leading cause of anaphylaxis (where the body shuts down and many people die) outside hospitals. Milk contributes to many of these reactions. [53] *As mentioned above, this has been my case.*

D) **More:** Interestingly enough, studies have proven that dairy products are also one of the leading factors in many other serious conditions such as irritable bowel syndrome (IBS), weak nutrient absorption, obesity and certain amino acid deficiencies.

E) **Cholesterol:** The cholesterol content of those three glasses of milk is equal to what one would get from 53 slices of bacon. Do you know of any doctor who recommends that much bacon per day? [54]

4.32   *Machiavellian Milk*

Imagine the following scene: You and your loved one (s) are driving down a country road and see cows meandering about in a farmers' field. You slam on the brakes and say, "Some cows! Honey! Let's go suckle (drink directly from the teat) the cows!" You all get out of the car trudge through the mud, get on your knees and begin suckling on the cows teats! Why is this so outlandish and really quite gross? The reason this is crazy is as *humans (and all other animals) we don't naturally crave drinking another animal's milk*. We don't even drink our own species' milk past the age of 2!). We drink milk and eat other dairy products conveniently avoiding the unpleasant parts of obtaining it! Do any other adult animals feed on a different animal's milk? Never! Think about it logically, a bovine calf goes from childhood to adulthood (from 90 pounds to 1000 pounds) in less than 1 year vs 21 years for a human to reach full growth. *The amount of pituitary hormone concentration required for this growth is much too high (even without the artificial hormones now fed to dairy cows).* This is one of the reasons goat's milk is preferred by vegetarians, anatomically, goats are much closer in size to humans and their milk contain less hormones as well as having natural anti-inflammatories that cow's milk lack. Goat's milk (and cheese) also does not require pasteurization leading many to believe it is a more natural and healthier choice. Almond Milk, Soy milk and rice milk are also great substitutes, try them all to find out which one (s) are your favorite(s)!

Only through a hundred years of marketing by powerful dairy boards have we (including myself!) been brainwashed with the phrase "Milk, it does the body good!" or "Got Milk?" and cute celebrity athlete milk mustaches or cartoon cows dancing! Not only does milk not "do the body good" it actually harms the body in many significant ways. The medical community and dieticians have also long told us (and often still minimize the risks), milk and other dairy products are good sources of calcium and fight degenerative diseases such as osteoporosis. *This is Fiction!* Fortunately, there are many better ways to get calcium than these high-fat, high protein, overly processed and hormone-laden white liquids. Many ads and associations (even some doctors) advocate a daily dose of dairy to ward off degenerative diseases such as osteoporosis which confuses the issue further. Thankfully many informed doctors (and almost every alternative health practitioner) now strongly discourage dairy.

4.33   *Calcium Consumption Conundrum*

The latest studies have conclusively shown that dairy products not only *do not help osteoporosis, they are one of the greatest causes of kidney problems, asthma, osteoporosis and cancer, yes cancer.* Much new literature finds that *cancer is consistently promoted by casein* (over 80% of cow's milk protein). Women who eat diets rich in animal foods excrete more calcium in their urine providing a negative calcium balance, a high risk factor for osteoporosis. This occurs because your body in its infinite wisdom leeches calcium from your bones to remove acidity (when there is no buffer: created by healthy diet).

"The calcium in cow's milk is basically useless because it has insufficient magnesium content (those nations with the highest amount of milk/dairy consumption also have the highest rates of osteoporosis). Need proof? How about a controlled study of 78,000 nurses over a period of 12 years?

Cows milk has three (3) times the calcium as does human breast milk. No matter, neither are very usable because in *order to be absorbed and used there MUST be an equal quantity of magnesium* (as exists in the greens that cows eat to get all the calcium they need for their big bones)." [55]

Building and maintaining bones is done with calcium. Other uses in the body include teeth, blood clotting, nervous impulse propagation and heart rhythm regulation. Over 98% of calcium in the human body is stored in our bones and teeth. The remaining small percent is in blood and tissue. The body gets calcium 2 ways: One is through eating calcium rich foods and the second way is by pulling it from the bones.

Eating animal protein (meat and dairy) increases the *acid load* on the body which makes the blood and tissues acidic. *To neutralize this acid, (remember in Section 3.4 the body will do anything to keep from being acidic) your body pulls calcium from the bones which weakens them.* A recent report published in the Journal of Pediatrics mentioned that boosting milk consumption or other *dairy products is not the best way* to provide the minimal 400 milligrams of calcium required per day.

"Calcium: Studies have shown that vegetarians absorb and retain more calcium from foods than do non-vegetarians. Vegetable greens such as spinach, kale and broccoli, and some legumes and soybean products are good sources of calcium from plants." [56]

4.34   *Osteoporosis Obstruction Options*

Osteoporosis is a bone disease with 3 characteristics: a) the amount of bone is decreased, b) the spongy interior of the bone is decreased and c) the surface of the bone gets thinner – rendering bones easily broken. Typical fractures occur in the spine, hips and wrists. These lead to chronic pain, impair mobility and can cause permanent disability. Recent estimates are that over 10 million Americans have osteoporosis and another 35 million have osteopenia, low bone mass leading to Osteoporosis. Both are responsible for over 1.5 million fractures annually. About half of women and a quarter of men are expected to get Osteoporosis in their lifetimes.

"American women have been consuming an average of 2 pounds of milk per day for their entire lives, yet 30 million American women have osteoporosis. Drinking milk does not prevent bone loss. Bone loss is accelerated by ingesting too much protein, and milk has been called "liquid meat."" [57]

Health Tip #27: The bad news: dairy destroys bone mass via calcium leaching, the good news: green leafy vegetables provide more than enough and don't leach any calcium from your bones. Osteoporosis does not need to happen as we age!

Opting Out of Osteoporosis:

Treatments are available but osteoporosis has no cure. *Prevention is therefore the key.* To minimize the risk as we age stay active, eat a variety of plant foods (especially dark green vegetables), avoid animal foods (and dairy) and reduce/eliminate salt intake. To guarantee you don't have problems perform regular weight-bearing exercises, consume the daily calcium amount (400 mg) and vitamin D (go outside!), avoid caffeine, alcohol and tobacco.

4.35   __Baby Bone Buster__

Children are often the targets of the powerful dairy industry and its lobbyists through focusing on schools and young mothers. Do kids who drink milk have stronger bones? A recent study in the Journal of Pediatrics states that thirty seven (37) studies examined the impact of calcium consumption on bone strength in children older than seven (7). Twenty seven (27) of these studies *did not support drinking more milk to boost calcium.* [58] Physical activity of youths was shown to be the primary stimulus for growth and development.

4.36   *__Lively Licensed Liquids__*

There are too many alternatives on the market today to continue to drink dairy milk. You don't have to give up your favorite foods to be healthy. Options include soy milk, rice milk, almond milk (my favorite!), yogurt made with rice or soy base, even sesame seed milk. Dairy foods *initially may appear* to contain more calcium in absolute amounts than calcium-rich plant foods. If absorption is taken into account, *the amount of plant food required to get the same amount of absorbable calcium is very small.* Examples:

1 Cup Cow's Milk	=	1 Cup of Soy Milk
	=	1 Cup of Kale/turnip greens
	=	0.7 cup of tofu
	=	1.7 cups of Broccoli [59]

One final thought around dairy products: The level of dairy product consumption in the US is one of the highest in the world (72% of calcium intake), and osteoporosis and fracture rates are also higher than any other country.

> *__Health Tip #27:__ The level of dairy product consumption in the US is one of the highest in the world (72% of calcium intake), and osteoporosis and fracture rates are also the highest.*

4.37 *Cheese, Ice Cream and Butter : Mega-Concentrated Milk*

Cheese and butter are much more concentrated than milk and are just as dangerous. Consider how much more concentrated these three foods are:

Product	Pounds of Milk to Make 1 Pound (454 grams) [60]
Cheese	10 lbs
Ice Cream	12 lbs
Butter	21 lbs

4.38 *Yogurt*

While there is relatively limited information on yogurt versus the other dairies (butter, milk and cheese), the main reason often given for consuming yogurt is the positive benefits in the intestinal tract: acidophilus flora being good for the gut. The following debunks this:

"In the mid-80's acidophilus was first suggested to have health benefits for humans. Acidophilus occurs naturally in the gastrointestinal tract but tends to grow slowly when added to milk (yogurt), leading to the risk of undesirable organisms. There is no direct proof and no consensus among researchers on whether or not added acidophilus in yogurt adheres to or colonizes in the intestines (3). Few human studies have been performed. A recent study reported that yogurt did not alter immunoglobulin secretions. *These results show no health benefits from yogurt consumption.*" [61]

The major problem with most yogurts is the sugars or sweeteners added. So if you must have yogurt get it as natural as possible (without flavorings) Overall, of all the dairies, yogurt seems to be the least offensive but should still be limited due to its provenance from the cow's milk (with all the casein and hormone concerns previously mentioned) until further study.

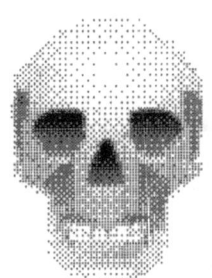

4.4   *Dinosore 4: Toxin 4 :*
An Acid Lifestyle

4.41   *Terrible Terrain*

As discussed in section 1.9 where we covered that the "terrain is everything", an acid lifestyle creates a terrain begging for future problems. Any diet that increases over-acidification of your blood system and tissues really makes your body an incredibly suitable terrain for an explosion of virus, bacteria and fungus. As covered earlier these are the *real enemy* that decompose (a more scientific word for kill!) the cells and tissues of your body.

A great analogy is the following. Think of a refrigerator which must stay cold for the food within it to stay fresh and free of bacteria, fungus and mold. If the terrain in the refrigerator is somehow corrupted (door is left open for an extended period, motor breaks etc.) and the fridge grows warmer. The food inside will begin to grow bacteria that evolve (mutate) into mold. Anyone who has kept a jar of salsa too long knows the green mold will be in the product! The food begins to deteriorate and is destroyed. *The same thing happens in your body when you over-eat acid-producing foods. This is how all infectious and degenerative diseases are created.*

Terminating the Terrain : Killing Fungus, Mold and Bacteria

So, now that we know the problem what's the solution? Again the solution may seem deceptively simple, but doesn't it make sense? Why complicate it: *Our bodies seek living, unadulterated foods.* To reduce and eliminate acid you must do what I have been suggesting throughout the book: *Eat living alkaline foods: dark green and yellow vegetables, sprouted nuts, soybeans, seeds, grains and essential fatty acids.* This diet will immediately lower the over-acidification of the blood and tissues with its huge quantity of bases and alkaline salts. As I am loath to keep saying, *don't take it from me*, try it in your body since you are your own expert!

> ***Health Tip #29: The solution to an acidic body:*** *Eat living alkaline foods: dark green and yellow vegetables, sprouted nuts, soybeans, seeds, grains and essential fatty acids.*

4.42   American (North) Acid Addiction

To stop the insanity of acid in your bloodstream and tissues *you must eliminate or dramatically reduce the following acid habits.*

1.   **Caffeine (includes Pop)**

2.   **Sugar (includes Pop)**

3.   **Nicotine**

4.   **Alcohol**

5.   **Whites**

6.   **Vinegar**

7.   **Drugs**

4.43   *#1 Acid Habit: Caffeine: Corner (Street) and Kitchen Consumption Catastrophe*

Perhaps the most underestimated destroyer of health is coffee. The alkaloid caffeine is the active ingredient in coffee, non-herbal tea, cocoa and soft drinks: *it is toxic, poison and a drug.* Unfortunately, western society is literally *addicted* to this drug. Coffee is the world's second most valuable commodity behind petroleum in terms of dollars. More than 500 million cups of coffee are ingested globally per year. The scary thing with coffee is how many people believe it is beneficial or harmless! My understanding and opinion is that *most of the coffee studies saying/ suggesting some version of "coffee is good for you" are subsidized by the remarkably powerful, global coffee cartels and lobbyists (similar to alcohol, food, pharmaceutical lobbyists).* Remember your first coffee? You were probably a jittery mess bouncing off the walls. Tea in general has 40 – 50mg of caffeine per cup. Green tea 20 to 30 mg. [62]

"Over half the population of the U.S. drinks at least two cups of coffee a day. Some 25% of coffee drinkers consume about five (5) cups daily, and another 25% drink ten (10) or more cups a day. Coffee is not just a beverage, it's a drug. Hundreds of thousands of law abiding citizens are physically addicted to coffee." [63]

4.44   *Coffee Collapse*

Caffeine *can never* be a part of a healthy and vital life since it severely weakens your body's vital life-giving forces.

1. Caffeine stimulates *(because your body is reacting violently to being poisoned!)* the adrenal (signifying on the kidney) glands to produce adrenaline and cortisone, hormones the human body depends on to raise heart rate, increase breathing as well as blood pressure. After years of this abuse, the adrenals become permanently *exhausted and stop responding.* This leaves you more vulnerable to a smorgasbord of health hazards.

2. *It can acutely impact the cardiovascular system* (high blood pressure, high cholesterol levels, arrhythmias or palpitations in the hearts of certain individuals). The digestive system including stomach upset, ulcers, diarrhea, reduced nutrient absorption, and energy expenditure.

3. *Coffee is a known carcinogen similar to nicotine.* There are hundreds of chemicals in coffee used in the roasting process, such as creosote and tar. There are some possible connections between caffeine and disease: bladder cancer in men, breast cancer in women and birth defects in pregnant women. If it is so safe and wonderful why can't pregnant women drink it like water? *I'll let you figure it out.*

4. *Other side-effects of the caffeine DRUG*: restlessness, anxiety, irritability, muscle tremors, sleeplessness, chronic fatigue, headaches, ulcers, etc.

When glucose levels in your body rise, the pancreas reacts strongly by releasing large amounts of insulin into the body. The sugar is then quickly used up as fuel this produces the "surge" in energy. Then the blood sugar level crashes giving people unpleasant symptoms such as headaches, unnecessary hunger and cravings, "the shakes" and fatigue. *As with all drugs, coffee creates an insatiable hunger for more and more!* Then if that wasn't enough, high insulin levels stop the release of growth hormones depressing your immune system. High insulin levels make the body "hungry" resulting in larger amounts storage in fat cells. Since most coffee is drank with dairy and sugar (not to mention all the lattes which are pure crème and sugar) these are 2 more reasons to eliminate it.

> **_Health Tip #30:_** *The Caffeine "boost" you get (which decreases with use over time) is actually your body's reaction of pumping adrenaline BECAUSE IT HAS BEEN POISONED.*

Source: U.S Food and Drug Administration and National Soft Drink Association 2004

Item	Quantity of Item	Average Amount of Caffeine
Coffee(drip)	5 ounces	115 mg
Iced Tea	12 ounces	70mg
Mountain Dew	12 ounces	55mg
Diet Coke	12 ounces	45mg
Coca-Cola	12 ounces	34mg
Cold Pill	1 tablet	30mg
Dark Chocolate	1 ounce	20mg
Milk Chocolate	1 ounce	6mg

I believe the biggest danger with coffee is the seeming cluelessness and love affair of most media and general population with coffee's dangers. Since so many are addicted no one notices the ship is sinking. *The trick to kick the coffee habit is to not do* it "cold turkey", big headaches will occur! Gradually decrease your coffee cups per day by half every 3 days. *Decaffeinated coffee is just as bad since the process uses Methylene Chloride, a powerful carcinogen.* If you must drive by and give the large multinationals some money towards their billions in revenue, order a herbal tea, they taste great. Some like mint or ginger are actually beneficial. Remember, coffee was invented thousands of years ago before anyone knew of its impact, similar to nicotine. In 40 or 50 years they will look back at how much damage we did to our bodies with this far from harmless beverage addiction. Consider yourself on the leading edge of knowing!

"A biochemist of my acquaintance says there's no way coffee would be legalized for sale as a food product if discovered today. *Might make it as an insecticide though.*"[64]

4.45 *#2 Acid Habit: Sugar: Sledgehammer Symphony*

Processed and refined sugars are toxic to you and *must be avoided* to maintain optimal health! Refined Sugar is very acidic and dramatically increases glucose levels in the blood very (too) quickly. Sugar is #1 on the list of items our good friends yeast, bacteria, mold and fungus feast on in your body. This "garbage in your garbage" is a perfect environment (terrain) for disease and nasty symptoms to arise. *As much as caffeine is a drug, sugar is also a drug!* It is generally known to cause diabetes, obesity, coronary thrombosis, tooth and gum decay, varicose veins (who knew!), stomach trouble and at least indirectly mental disturbances.

What do you think is the most common source of sugar in our diets? Desserts and sweets? No and no! Soft Drinks which have increased 500% in consumption from the 1950's to today. More than 50 million cola beverages are consumed daily in the US! According to the National Soft Drink Association *the average 12-ounce (355 ml) regular (non-diet), carbonated soft drinks contains the equivalent of 10 teaspoons of sugar and 150 calories.* This colossal amount of sugar *literally immobilizes the immune system* by about 1/3. Three (3) cans of soft drinks a day will shut down your immune system for an entire day. *Gentlemen: Another nasty side-effect of soft drinks is erectile dysfunction.*

"Are you looking for effective home remedies for *erectile dysfunction?* ... Avoid *soft drinks* and coffee..." [65]

One study reported in Journal of the American Medical Association (JAMA) of Aug. 2005 [66] suggests that a woman who consumes just one can of a soft drink a day is *83% more likely to get diabetes* than one who has less than one can a month.

Health Tip #31: If you must drink a soft drink, drink 7-UP or Diet 7-UP, Sprite or Diet Sprite and Sierra Mist all have no caffeine and the diet ones have only trace amounts of sugar. Ginger ales also have no caffeine.

If the above hasn't convinced you, try this. The estrogen-mimicking chemical BPA, which has already been banished from water jugs and baby bottles has shown up in significant levels in soft drinks and energy drinks tested by Health Canada. [67]

4.46 *Drink Destruction Data !*

Source: University of Cincinati Biology [68]

Soft Drink	Amount of Sugar
Diet 7-UP	0.16 teaspoon (tsp)
Diet Pepsi	1.96 tsp
Coke, Classic	9.15 tsp
Pepsi	9.5 tsp
Mountain Dew	10.47 tsp
Dr. Pepper	19.17 tsp
Diet Coke	33.67 tsp
A&W Root Beer	110.25 tsp (This = 2.3 cups of sugar!)

4.47 *Diet Drink Dilemma*

A note on diet soft drinks, they may not have much sugar but the chemicals are often worse and have unknown effects on growing children.

"But in my experience, it's actually a wolf in sheep's clothing, fooling women into thinking they are doing something good for their bodies when they are actually sabotaging their own best efforts. Diet soda may not have the sugar or calories of regular soda, but it's chock-full of other health-draining chemicals, like *caffeine, artificial sweeteners, sodium and phosphoric acid.* This is even more concerning when parents give their *growing — and chemically vulnerable —* children diet soda in a noble effort to avoid sugar." [69]

Many new studies also show an increased risk of obesity correlated to diet soft drinks.

4.48 *Juggling Juice Jugs*

Read Labels on juices since they are hugely sugary! Some so-called "natural" juices can contain up to 5 teaspoons of sugar per serving! According to the Oklahoma Fit Kids Coalition [70] ; a school-age child in Oklahoma, on average, drinks 4 x 12 ounce (355 ml) of soft drinks per day. I figure statistics are similar elsewhere. Children who are sedentary (inactive or under-active) and who drink that much pop per day *will gain a staggering 13 pounds a year. Here's a sobering fact, to burn the calories from 4 cans of pop, your child would have to ride a bike for 4 hours!*

4.49 *Sugar Creates Acid → Acid Creates Glue*

Many people believe sugar causes cavities, not directly. The sugar turns into acid which causes cavities. If the acid is strong enough to burn through the one of the hardest elements known to man, tooth enamel, (for an idea of how powerful acid is: when a body is burnt to a crisp in a fire, dental remains are all that are left!). Think of what it does to your soft tissues inside your body! *Sugar turns into acid which turns into glue in your body.* This glue gums up your blood which causes heart attacks, strokes and basically creates a perfect terrain for disease. Similarly, "concentrated" cans of juice (orange, apple, etc.) have been heat-treated and are acidic.

Health Tip #32: Sugar turns to acid powerful enough to cut through tooth enamel (cavities) the hardest human body part, think of what it does to soft tissues inside you! It turns into glue.

4.49   *Energy Drinks: Elixir Euphoria (Not!)*

One last area of concern is this issue of *energy drinks* (Monster, Red Bull etc.). They are all the rage especially amongst the late teens and early adults. I would like to be on record as saying these drinks are analogous to putting rocket fuel in your average car. Sure it will go faster for awhile but at what cost? Most of these energy drinks have the equivalent of one cup's worth of coffee which we have already discussed. Then they add in all these jazzy eastern-sounding herbs such as Taurine, Guarana, Ginko Biloba, Ginseng, etc. *They are not regulated* as regular foods are either. Add in a truckload of sugar (in general similar to pop, about 12 teaspoons of sugar per can) and you have a real time bomb, literally. Many young people add in alcohol to these already dehydrating drinks which is quite frightening. The bottom line is there are very few studies on energy drinks yet but the initial information we have seems problematic.

"My main concern with the use of the herbs in these drinks is their source. The mass manufacturers of energy drinks are not required by law to list whether or not the herbs they use, have been sprayed with toxic pesticides, irradiated or watered with contaminated water supplies, so there is no telling what other toxins are contained in these drinks and whether or not these herbs will have a negative effect on the body." [71]

4.50   *Soft Drink Suggestions and Substitutes*

To help you from completely going cold turkey on soft drinks here are some suggestions that worked for myself and others I know who have kicked (or seriously decreased) the habit.

1. When drinking a can of pop drink only 1/3 to ½ the can and throw the rest away or split it with someone (right here you can decrease your intake 50% to 66%).

2. Drink 2 large glasses of water 30 minutes before a meal, you won't be as thirsty and can avoid pop.

3. Use sparkling water with lime or lemon or a mix of ½ orange or apple juice and ½ sparkling water. (I don't necessarily recommend sparkling water as it contains a significant amount of sodium).

4. At restaurants, always start drinking your water with lemon and lime, then pop until you kick the habit.

5. Use them at group celebrations, never buy it for the house, you can't drink what's not there!

4.51 *Acid Habit #3: Nefarious, Needless and Nasty Nicotine*

I won't spend much time on this one because basically the cat's out of the bag on cigarette/cigar/pipe smoking and nicotine (it took a long time as the lobbyists were powerful swearing up and down nicotine was not a health hazard). The food and drug lobbyists are where the cigarette companies were 30 and 20 years ago, in 20 years hopefully we will look back at this time as the "dark ages" for food! The negative effects are widely well known. They are listed on the packages! Risks include asthma, heart disease, stroke, lung cancer, emphysema and hypertension. Smoking caused more than 168,000 deaths in 2005.[72] Smoking has one difference vs all other toxins mentioned before: *You can injure others by smoking too.* I don't know too many foods that are toxic to others when you eat them (maybe an egg salad sandwich!). Bottom line, if you are reading this you care enough about your health to know this one. Marijuana, pipes and cigars are also smoking!

Health Tip #33: There is no possibility for any semblance of medium or long term health or vitality while consuming cigarettes or even a few drinks of alcohol per week. Choose, but know and accept your role in the consequences. It's your choice and your body, no one else's.

4.52 *Acid Habit #4: Alcohol as an Asinine Act*

Do you know how powerful the alcohol lobbyists and industry are? Think massive, global, hugely powerful entities with very deep pockets and connections. Realize that many if not most of the stories written or studies completed on the medicinal positive effects of "one alcoholic drink a day" have been sponsored by the powerful alcohol companies or associations. Wine growing and alcohol trading associations are as powerful as the coffee growers associations and have clout and influence beyond our comprehension. *Alcohol is a depressant.* We all know the effects of alcoholism, but what about the rather large contingent who drink a few drinks per week? They generally feel they are ok since almost everyone shares the same destructive habit. If you feel you need a few drinks to "warm up" or "be smooth" you might want to start doing some internal work on yourself, i.e. consider yoga, martial arts, taking classes, anything that challenges you and gets you to a place where you don't require stimulants or depressants to have a good time. Having a good time without chemicals really shows integration as a human to enjoy living for what it is, a wonderful moment by moment privilege. If you have ever had a major injury or hospitalization you remember how great it felt to be well again. As humans we often forget what we have until we lose it.

Boozy Brain Drain

One drink of 1 ounce of alcohol kills *thousands of brain cells and permanently damages the brain.* The liver is already overburdened with our acid lifestyle, we add another acid?!?!

"The researchers suggested blood thickening, even in social drinkers, may be sufficient to block fine blood pathways in the brain and cause brain damage. Alcohol's inhibition of brain activity also affects vision. At a blood-alcohol concentration of around 0.08 per cent, the eyes' ability to focus is disturbed to such an extent that depth vision is impeded and double vision may occur. There is also evidence higher blood alcohol levels may be risk factors in night blindness and cataracts. They suggest *mild brain damage* is so common that it affects the performance of many (among others) police, politicians and bureaucrats. Further evidence that even moderate drinking damages the brain comes from recent (2004) studies at Johns Hopkins University." [73]

The media via the wine growers do an excellent job convincing us that a drink of wine per day is healthy. They point to the Mediterranean diet where populations age with much less risk of heart attack, cancer or stroke. The key thing in the Mediterranean diet that allows people to live healthier and longer *is the amount of organic fresh fruits and vegetables they eat.* They walk or bicycle everywhere. Meat is a small part of most of their dishes and they have more fish. They use olive oil and canola oil and living herbs copiously (plants such as basil and oregano). Produce is fresh from the market. They drink water instead of soft drinks, small quantities of nuts and figs. Their coffees are strong but small (1 ounce). They eat whole wheat breads without butter or margarine, etc. etc.

"For example, residents of Greece eat very little red meat and average nine (9) servings a day of antioxidant-rich fruits and vegetables. The Mediterranean diet has been associated with a lower level of oxidized low-density lipoprotein (LDL) cholesterol — the "bad" cholesterol that's more likely to build up deposits in your arteries." [74]

So the ***alcohol is not why*** the Mediterranean diet is so healthy.

__Health Tip #34:__ Wine (and alcohol) __IS NOT__ the healthy aspect of the Mediterranean Diet, it is the focus on fresh produce, little meat and fish with little hydrogenised fat.

4.53   *Acid Habit #5: Woeful Whites*

Whites can be defined as all processed products devoid of life and nutrition. This includes but is not limited to:

Wheat products (Bread and Pasta)

Breads

Rice

Sugar

Potatoes (white)

Any bleached, roasted nuts (peanuts, almonds)

It's a good practice to avoid the above foods because they are all are very high in carbohydrates and have high glycemic indexes (they cause blood sugar levels to spike up uncontrollably then crash).

Another concern: Did you know stored grains (wheat, rice, barley) begin to ferment in 90 days in normal conditions creating an environment saturated with mytotoxins? Although a natural process, it can't be prevented. Corn and peanuts are easily contaminated with fungi.

Substitutes: If you must eat wheat, get organic spelt, whole grain wheat breads, brown or wild rices. Use sweet potatoes (high beta carotene) instead of potatoes, even as fries in some restaurants!

Some great grains: Barley, Bran. Brown rice, Buckwheat, Bulgur, cornmeal, Hominy, Oats, Quinoa, cracked wheat, wheat germ and wild rice. Get unprocessed California Almonds.

> *__Health Tip #35:__ Eliminate "white" breads, pasta, rices, nuts. Replace with Barley, Bran. Brown rice, Buckwheat, Bulgur, cornmeal, Hominy, Oats, Quinoa, cracked wheat, wheat germ and wild rice.*

4.54 *Acid Habit #6: Vicious Vinegar*

All pickled products are in a jar, beets, pickles, olives, etc. White vinegar on fries and vinegar in salad dressings. Vinegar is a product of decay; it comes from a double fermentation of sugar first to alcohol (yeasts and fungus) and a second fermentation to vinegar. So Sugar then fungus makes alcohol, more fungus makes vinegar. It can't be good for the body. Vinegar's main problem is acetic acid which attacks the liver and brain in much the same way as alcohol does. Vinegar actually *thickens* your blood. This puts a strain on the heart and interferes with the digestion of starches. Before fully going cold turkey on salad dressing, try this great hint to use less. Ask for dressing on the side and you dip your fork in it before every bite. You will be amazed! You will use about 60% to 70% less salad dressing. To replace salad dressing fully; use olive oil, lemon and garlic.

4.55 *Acid Habit #7: Pharmaceutical Folly*

Did you know *Americans spent the same amount on pharmaceuticals (over $250 Billion in 2005) the same as they do on gasoline!* The dangers of illegal drugs are well documented and publicized. The potential deadly effects of prescription drugs are rarely fully illustrated and explained. We live in a quick fix, "fast food solution" society. We look for quick solutions to problems we have created in ourselves over decades of abuse through the genius of modern chemistry. Billions of dollars are spent by pharmaceutical companies annually in marketing their particular "magic bullet" prescription drugs to consumers. Luckily, common sense is beginning to permeate consumers as unsafe drugs are removed from sale after disastrous side effects or complications. For example Vioxx was rapidly pulled off the market after it was found to *double the risk of heart attack and stroke* in users. That being the case, Americans purchase more medicine per person than residents of every other nation. About 130 million of them swallow, inject, inhale, infuse, spray and rub drugs from 3.5 Million prescriptions written each year.

Over-the-Counter drugs should not be considered 100% reliable or safe. One drug, (naproxen) also known as Aleve made headlines when it was linked to a 50% increase in heart attacks. Readily available painkillers can create stomach irritation/bleeding. Some allergy medications have side effects such as irregular heartbeat.

> *Health Tip #36: Taking care of your health first allows you more choice physically, spiritually and financially! Risking your health is literally financial suicide. If you are in a relationship, get and stay fit together!*

4.6 *A Healthy Physical Environment Outside your Body*

Now that you've made it this far, you have all the information to have a powerful, long-term sustainable knowledge foundation for taking charge of your health, energy and vitality. With this (hopefully) strong internal base in place you're ready for any curveballs the world and life might throw at you. You must and will continue to grow in terms of health, *the most important area of your life.* In this last section, I would like to offer you a few tips for you to sustain and improve your home environment. Our modern world has become a hazard to our health in terms of the number of chemicals used in so many areas for cost savings and convenience. There are today many options to "go natural" in your life fostering more long term resilience to disease. Here are a few areas to get the ball rolling (I'm sure you will discover more, let me know your suggestions!).

1) **Cosmetics: Protect your skin!**
2) **Chlorine: Shower Safety**
3) **Cleaning Products: Toxic Minefield**
4) **Dry Cleaning challenges**
5) **Commercial Beverages**
6) **Protecting the air you breathe**

4.61 *Corrosive Cosmetics*

Undoubtedly, one of the most common, yet least understood sources of toxicity in our bodies comes from the many modern toiletries and cosmetics we use on a daily basis. Without giving it a second thought, most people are either ingesting or absorbing through their skin a myriad variety of toxicity via chemicals. Thankfully we now have many clean sources for these types of products, products that are neutral or positive for you and our mother earth.

Aluminum appears to be one of the worst culprits, it is found in most commercial antiperspirants and deodorants. It is suspected to cause a major role in Alzheimer's disease, only one of many forms of dementia impacting up to 10% of all people over 65. These persons have been reported to have up to 4X the normal concentration of aluminum in the cells of their brains. Aluminum also is a known neurotoxin that can cause brain damage in large exposure amounts.

"These compounds are very soluble and are readily absorbed by the body. Once in the body, the aluminum portion of the molecule ionizes, forming free radical aluminum (Al+++). This passes freely across cell membranes and forms a physical plug, that when dissolved is selectively absorbed by the liver, kidney, brain, cartilage and bone marrow. It is this concentration of aluminum that has been the source for concern in the medical community, and has prompted the research being done on Alzheimer's disease and Breast Cancer victims. The human body has a few areas that it uses to purge toxins: Behind the knees, ears, groin area and armpits." [75]

Antiperspirants stop the body from perspiring in the armpit area, this causes your body to deposit them in the lymph nodes since it can't sweat them out. This causes high concentrations of toxins which lead to cell mutations which can cause cancer. If my understanding is correct, *nearly all breast cancer tumors occur in the upper outside area where the lymph nodes reside.* Even if this is 50% true, why risk it?

Health Tip #37: When you shower, you are exposed to twenty (20) times the amount of chlorine and toxic chemicals than from drinking regular chlorinated tap water.

4.62   *Chlorine Challenge*

Most of us realize the dangers of chlorinated water in the water we drink and choose purified/filtered water. What about the water you shower with, clean dishes with or do laundry with? Did you know that when you shower, you are exposed to 20 times the amount of chlorine and toxic chemicals than from just drinking tap water. The best solution (one I will implement) is to buy a filter for your shower, laundry and dishwashing water. There are many fine providers of filtration systems. Search the internet.

4.63   *House Cleaning: Cleaning or Carcinogen?*

Just as important as the cosmetics going on your skin are the household cleansers you use. These include dishwasher soap, laundry detergent, glass, counter and floor cleaners. When commercial products are used, toxic chemicals are released into the air you breathe, clothes you wear, etc. There are a variety of companies today that produce all natural, environmental-friendly products for home use. You can find some in local health-food stores.

Health Tip #38: *Find natural and mild cleaners for the home.*

4.64   *Dry Cleaning Disaster*

Dry cleaners have traditionally used a chemical called perchloroethylene or "perc" for short. This chemical is toxic and has been showing harmful effects on the nervous system and all major organs. This chemical has caused dizziness, respiratory issues, nervous system challenges, reproductive disorders as well as higher cancer risks. The International Agency for Research in Cancer (IARC) classifies perc as a "probable human carcinogen". Many modern stores don't use the chemical, look for "wet cleaning" or "no perc" signs at dry cleaners. An EPA study revealed that bringing fresh dry cleaning into your house can result in perc levels exceeding the guidelines. Some washing machines clean at a high temperature allowing for deeper cleaning of clothes. Here's a trick I use for shirts. I wash them normally then once they are clean put them in the dryer for 10 minutes only, once done put them immediately on a hanger. Shirts will be crisp and look dry cleaned (ensure shirts are on pleats on hangers). Also available today are "no dry clean required" shirts. If you must continue to dry clean your clothes, remove them from the bag as soon as you get home and hang them outside or a well ventilated area.

__Health Tip #39__: In terms of dry cleaning look for "no perc" process to reduce cancer risk.

4.65   *Indoor Issues*

You should take some precautions around the air in your home. Indoor air quality has been said to be up to 25% to 60% more dangerous than outdoor air quality. Some suggestions for the home include the following:

- Ensure the oven ventilation goes to the outside of your home.

- Open windows when cleaning and vacuuming your home

- Have your air ducts cleaned regularly.

- Clean your washroom fans regularly.

- Anything that creates smoke in your home is a hazard, from fireplaces to cigarettes should be eliminated.

- Avoid using toxic floor cleaners, Murphy's Oil or Pine Sol are good choices

"We do not inherit the earth from our ancestors, we borrow it."
Native American Proverb

6.0   <u>Your Commitment To Health</u>

So this is gut-check time, you have enough (more than) information and tools to change your habits and begin living a vibrant, full, and energetic, healthy life *without fear!* You're ready to feel how great it is to be optimally healthy – *at any stage*. You're ready to implement these strategies into your daily plan, congratulations! The bigger issue here is: *how committed are you to your health?* The difference between being "on a diet" and "making a lifestyle choice" are as different as they can be. If you are committed to your health you will know when to choose health over popularity, health over convenience or cost. That's what it will take to be committed no matter where you are or the people you are with. *The 40 day Challenge is your opportunity to recreate and reframe who you are physically, emotionally and spiritually.* Hopefully exercise becomes your drug, vitality your habit. Health is the rule not the exception. Your coach potato days are over, you're a gym rat, a health fiend, an example for others of what is possible in terms of health! Congratulations! Here are some questions to ask yourself:

What is *my new identity* around full energy and vitality?

Why is this important to me? *(What is the purpose of this? The "why I'm doing this is…")*

How committed am I to this, there will be bumps, you must keep your eyes on the goal/prize!

What are some of the huge actions you will take immediately to lock it in? Join a gym? Throw out all your junk food? Buy a vegan recipe book? Go to a health food store? Hire a health coach/trainer? *Do it now! Never leave the scene of a choice or decision without taking action immediately.*

Who will support me in this journey? Who will hold me to this? Who can do this with me?

<u>Remember:</u> It takes 28 to 40 days to create a new habit. Hang in there!

> ***Health Tip #40:*** *It is of utmost importance to be committed to your health for the rest of your life, all other decisions are secondary to this.*

6.1 Implementation: 40 Tips For 40 Days : The 40 Day Plan

So, now you're committed! Good for you! Here is the plan for the next 40 days. *Stick to it, be your word with yourself.* You can't do this and feel any appreciable difference in your body unless you allow the 40 day time window its impact on your body.

The 40 Day Plan:

1. *Breathing and Lymphasizing*

   a) Take 10 Deep Breaths 3 times a day.

   b) Do 20-30 minutes of rebounding every day.

2. *Live Water and Fresh Live Foods*

   a) Drink 50% of your body weight in ounces of water per day

   b) Find a pure source of water

   c) Ensure your diet is 70% water-rich foods (aka: produce)

3. *Essential Oils*

Supplement food with Essential Fatty Acids (Omega 3's and 6's) your body needs.

   a) Eat foods that contain unadulterated and unprocessed *natural fats* in their original state: Examples include avocado, nuts such as almonds, hazelnuts, pumpkin and sunflower seeds. Oils such as flax seed, olive oil, fish oil or Udo's Blend Oil (or equivalent).

4. ***Alkalinity: Power Greens***

   a) Eat 70% (or more!) foods that create alkalinity and give life to your body. These include green and yellow vegetables, avocados, bananas, tomatoes, lemons, etc.

   b) *Eliminate* acid-creating foods that are dead, or worse dead and fried or dead and chemical-laden. This includes animal flesh, dairy (less yogurt), refined white foods, fried foods, sugars, caffeine.

   c) Lemon or lime in water.

   d) Supplement with a super-concentrated green drink to stay alkaline.

   e) Test your pH daily to monitor.

5. ***Aerobic Energy & Strength***

   a) Ensure you have a powerful base with 30 minutes of quality aerobic exercise a minimum of a minimum of 3 up to 5 times a week. Ideas include walking (get a dog!), running, swimming, aerobics, spinning or yoga class, skiing, snowboarding, etc. This will lower your set point.

   b) Stay in aerobic range of training, calculated as 180- your age.

   c) Create or get help in creating a training plan, keep challenging yourself.

   d) Have fun! Add different things to the mix such as friends, music, a change of environment, a race and many others. This will keep it fresh.

6. ***Peak Nourishment***

   a) ***Follow the rules to healthy eating:***

      i) Drink water 30 minutes before or after your meals, not during.

    ii) Combine foods properly:

        Eat fruit only on an empty stomach (not with other foods),

        Never eat protein and carbohydrates together,

        Eat green vegetables/salads with proteins or carbohydrates

        Never combine fats with proteins

        If you eat meats, eat them at lunch

    iii) Always eat in a relaxed state.

    iv) Eat comfortable amounts of food, allowing you to live longer and eat more!

    v) As much as feasible: eat organic (foods free of pesticides, antibiotics and hormones).

  b Watch for sugar overloads.

  c) **Follow the food pyramid:** 70% live foods, 10% plant-based proteins or fish, 10% carbohydrates and 10% quality oils.

  d) Supplements

    i) Wheatgrass, Digestive Enzymes, Oils, Acidophilus, Anti-oxidants, liquid multivitamins and condition specific supplements.

    ii) Periodic cleansing

    iii) Reward yourself for success

7. *__Alignment & Power__*

  a) **Keep Moving!** Make it a point to not stagnate, stay active, take the stairs, park far.

  b) **Ensure proper alignment and stretch regularly.** See an osteopath or chiropractor to ensure alignment and no pinching.

8. *Mindset*

   a) **Manage the runaway toxic thought patterns:** Ensure your mindset and inner dialogue is empowering and motivating. Primary focus on gratitude, courage, faith, determination, compassion and love.

   b) **Focus on your heart breathing**

   c) **Do a mind hurricane of Positive Emotional Hurricane 5 minutes a day.**

Eliminate the 4 Toxins From Your Life

9. *Toxin 1 :Remove or Drastically Decrease Intake of Processed Fats*

   a) Eliminate or dramatically reduce your consumption of all 1) processed fats, 2) trans fats, 3) hydrogenated fats.

   b) *Keep total fat intake below 25%, ideally 10%*

10. *Toxin 2: Eliminate or Drastically Decrease Animal Flesh*

    a) Eliminate or drastically reduce your animal flesh consumption

    b) Keep your protein to 5-6% of your intake and should come from plants which are more efficient, have more antioxidants, fiber and minerals.

    c) At least go 10 days without all animal meat (fish is ok). If after that period you still feel like consuming it follow the rules: i) eat it maximum once a day, ii) combine it with green vegetables and salad, eat it mid-day, choose from a free range, kosher, antibiotic free and organic source.

11. *Toxin 3: Eliminate or Drastically Decrease Dairy Consumption*

    a) *Toss all cow dairy products and sample the wonderful almond, soy and rice alternatives.* They taste phenomenal and have great texture.

b) *Calcium intake daily should be 400 milligrams per day and should be from plant sources which are calcium rich.* Remember that cow's milk leeches calcium from your bones.

12. *Toxin Close the Door on Your Acid Lifestyle*

a) Acids are the problem, get rid of them.

b) Say no to *caffeine, sugar, whites, vinegar, alcohol, nicotine and drugs (illicit and prescription). Really try 40 days without them and see the great energy and vitality you are missing with these.*

c) **Stay Alkaline:** When you are eating 70% to 80% life-giving and alkaline foods. Your body will naturally stop craving these addictions. Take a green drink

6.2 *Summary*

So we have covered so much ground! I want to congratulate you on hanging in there. Hopefully you enjoyed this book, my first book (hi mom!). You *are the only one in control of your life* and your health. *Your greatest strength is to maintain responsibility for how you feel, don't blame anyone else! Don't give up responsibility* for the most important and most far-reaching aspect of your life. Spend the time on exercise it's so much better than waiting in hospital or emergency rooms. Don't be a statistic, be one of those who sets the standard for what someone of your age looks, feels, acts and does! If this book has awakened huge curiosity about the many ideas I have presented, I have included a reading list. Congratulations on making to the end! You have the tools, make your health a life project, I am convinced it and you are so worth it! I have included in the next session some readings you may be interested in if this book sparked you! If you want to contact me, please email me at frank@myquantumleapcoaching.ca or visit my webpage at www. quantumleapcoaching.blogspot.com. I'd love to hear from anyone with comments on *Killing Yourself With Your Fork?* Let me also know about your successes and challenges with the 40 Day Plan! May all the health and vitality be yours! Live passionately!

6.3   Recommended Supplemental Readings

Fast Food Nation – The Dark Side of the All-American Meal by Eric Sclosser

Fit For Life by Harvey and Marilyn Diamond

Mad Cow Howard F. Lyman with Glen Merzer

Milk – The Deadly Poison by Robert Cohen

Natural Cures "They" Don't Want You to Know About by Kevin Trudeau

Power Aging by Gary Null, Ph.D

Slaughterhouse by Gail A. Eisnitz

The Amazing Liver Cleanse by Andreas Moritz

The Calcium Factor: The Scientific Secret of Health and Youth by Robert R. Barefoot and Carl J. Reich, M.D.

The Healing of Cancer – The Cures – the Cover-ups and the Solution Now by Berry Lynes

The pH Miracle by Robert O. Young, Ph.D and Shelley Redford Young

Your Body's Many Cries For Water by F. Batmanghelidj, M.D.

Your Drug May Be Your Problem by Peter R. Breggin, M.D.

6.4   Endnotes

1   Unleash The Power Within, viewed 2 November, 2009, http://www.tonyrobbins.com/UPWEvents/upwEnroll_Live.aspx

2   www.jacklalanne.com/jack.html   Jack   Lalanne,   viewed   12 December, 2008,

3   www.thebucketlist.warnerbros.com, 2007

4   www.wisegeek.com/what-is-the-krebs-cycle.htm   Dubroff,   Dee, "What Is The Krebs Cycle", viewed 30 November, 2008

5   Stanley L. Robbins, MD. Professor of Pathology, Harvard Medical School

6   "My 'Cure' for the common cold (and flu), http://www.healityourself.com/articlelive/articles/26/1/My-Cure-for-the-Common-Cold-and-Flu/Page1.html

7   NCHS Vital Statistics System for numbers of deaths, Bureau of Census for population estimates. Statistics compiled by the Office of Statistics and Programming, NCIPC, CDC., 1997

8   Flower, Samantha, "Bechamp & Pasteur – Clash & Consequence", viewed 15 November, 2008, http://www.samanthaflower.co.uk/phdi/p1.nsf/pages/1080:PDF_Bechamp_Pasteur.pdf/$file/PDF_Bechamp_Pasteur.pdf

9   Discoveries   and   Breakthroughs   Inside   Science,   Termite Terminator: "Why Do Termites Eat Wood?", February 1, 2004, viewed November 28, 2008, http://www.aip.org/dbis/stories/2004/14110.html

10 Weil, Andrew, viewed December 24, 2008, http://www.drweil.com/

11 Trudeau, Kevin, "How to Lose Weight Effortlessly and Keep It Off)!!", Pg. 163

12 Dr. F. Batmanghelidj, viewed 20 November 2008, http://www. watercure.com/

14 "Coffee_Linked_to_Adrenal_Gland_Disorders", originally on http://ping.sg/user/nocaf4me blog, 7 December, 2007, viewed 8 December, 2008, http://www.flixya.com/blog/NoCaf4Me/0/ Health,%20Food,%20Coffee,%20Nutrition

15 Pravda, 21 July, 2006, viewed 6 December, 2008, http://english. pravda.ru/science/health/83458-1/

16 16. http://survivalacres.com/information/water_content.html

17 Smith, Thomas, "Insulin: Our Silent Killer", viewed 3 December, 2008, http://www.shirleys-wellness-cafe.com/flaxoil.htm

18 Udo Erasmus, Ph.D, viewed 17 November, 2008, www. udoerasmus.com

19 "Acid-Alkaline Balance", http://www.naturalhealthschool.com/ acid-alkaline.html

20 Avalon Wolfe, Frankie, "The Complete Idiot's Guide to Being Vegetarian", 2nd edition, page 72, Viewed, 1 December, 2008, Alpha Books, ISBN 002863950-2 22.

21 Young, Dr. Robert O. & Young, Shelley Redford, "The pH Miracle", AOL Time Warner Books, viewed 23 November, 2008, http://www.phmiracleliving.com/c-25-books-dvds-audios.aspx

22 Viewed 12 December, 2008, http://www.bobdelmonteque.com/

23 "Exercise Proves valuable in Lowering Risk for Alzheimer's and Parkinson's", Senior Journal, 15 March, 2005, viewed 12 December, 2008, http://seniorjournal.com/NEWS/Health/5-03-15Alzheimers-Parkinsons.htm

24 2005 Stein, Rob, "Exercise Can Cut Risk of Dying From Breast Cancer", Washington Post, 25 May, 2005, viewed 11 December, 2008, http://www.washingtonpost.com/wp-dyn/content/article/2005/05/24/AR2005052401027.html

25 Better Health channel, "Fatigue Fighting Tips", 7/15/2004, viewed 12 Novemebr, 2008 http://www2.betterhealth.vic.gov.au/bhcgsearch/bhcgsearch?start=0&searchtext=Fatigue+Fighting+Tips

26 Garber, Carol Ewing, PhD, Associate Professor of cardiopulmonary and exercise science at the Bouve College of Health Sciences at Northeastern University in Boston. Brigham and Women's Hospital Health Information

27 Garber, Carol Ewing, PhD, Associate Professor of cardiopulmonary and exercise science at the Bouve College of Health Sciences at Northeastern University in Boston. Brigham and Women's Hospital Health Information

28 Workout IQ Web page, viewed 11 December, 2008, http://workoutiq.com/blog/2008/09/21/the-metabolic-setpoint

29 Paige Waehner, About.com:Exercise, "How Many calories Does Muscle Really Burn?", May 17, 2006, http://exercise.about.com/od/exerciseworkouts/f/muscle.htm

30 Shelton, Herbert, M.D. "Food Combining Made Easy", Herbert Shelton, M.D.

31 N. Phillip Norman, M.D., Adjunct Professor of Stomatology, Lecturer in Gastroenterology, New York Polyclinic medical School and Hospital

32 Fletcher, Robert H. , MD,MSc; Fairfield, Kathleen M. MD,DrPH, "Vitamins for Chronic Disease Prevention in Adults" Journal of the American Medical Association, 19 June 2002, http://jama.ama-assn.org/cgi/content/abstract/287/23/3127

33 Egoscue Method Clinic, San Diego, California, www.egoscue.com

34 Childre, Doc Lew, Martin, Howard, beech, Donna, Institute of Heartmath, "The Heartmath Solution, 1999, Harper Collins, http:harpercollins.com

35 Childre, Doc Lew, Martin, Howard, beech, Donna, Institute of Heartmath, "The Heartmath Solution, 1999, Harper Collins, http:harpercollins.com

36 http://www.palmoiltruthfoundation.com, viewed 4 November, 2008, http://www.palmoiltruthfoundation.com/index. php?option=com_search&Itemid=62&searchword=trans+fats+d ouble+&searchphrase=any&ordering=newest

37 Spurlock, Morgan, Supersize Me, 2004

38 U.S Department of Agriculture, 1999, USDA Nutrient Database for Standard Reference

39 Robbins, John, "The Food Revolution: How Your Diet Can Help Save Your Life and Our World", Pg. 421, Conari Press Books, 2001, conari.com

40 Campbell, T. Collin, PhD., Campbell II, Thomas M., "The China Study: Startling Implications for Diet, Weight Loss and Long-Term Health", BenBella Books, http://www.thechinastudy.com/buy.html

41 Julia E Klein-Geltink, Bernard CK Choi and Richard N Fry, "Chronic Diseases in Canada", Volume 27, No. 1, 2006, viewed 23 January, 2009, http://www.phac-aspc.gc.ca/publicat/cdic-mcc/27-1/index.html

42 Julia E Klein-Geltink, Bernard CK Choi and Richard N Fry, "Chronic Diseases in Canada", Volume 27, No. 1, 2006, viewed 23 January, 2009, http://www.phac-aspc.gc.ca/publicat/cdic-mcc/27-1/index.html

43 Brody, Jane E., "As America Gets Bigger the World Does Too.", The New York Times April 19, 2005, viewed 12 January, 2009, http://www.nytimes.com/2005/04/19/health/nutrition/19obes. html

44 "Canadian Beef Banned Too", viewed 12 January, 2009, http://www.mad-cow.org/~tom/ban_on_US_beef.html

45 Cancer Prevention Coalition, "American Beef, Why is it Banned in Europe?", http://www.preventcancer.com/consumers/general/hormones_meat.htm

46 PBS Frontline, viewed 12 january, 2009, http://www.pbs.org/wgbh/pages/frontline/shows/meat/safe/overview.html

47 Avalon Wolfe, Frankie, "The Complete Idiot's Guide to Being Vegetarian", 2nd edition, page 88, Viewed, 1 December, 2008, Alpha Books, ISBN 002863950-2 22.

48 Catherine Caulfield, "A Reporter at Large: The Rain Forests." New Yorker, January 14, 1985,

49 Website of EarthSave International, viewed 13 January, 2009, http://www.earthsave.org/pdf/summer2002.pdf

50 Website of EarthSave International, viewed 13 January, 2009, http://www.earthsave.org/pdf/summer2002.pdf

51 Lyman, Howard F. "Mad Cowboy", Touchstone 1998, page 23.

52 Adams, Mike, Natural News.com, viewed 23 January, 2009, http://www.naturalnews.com/011148.html

53 Bykowski, Mike,"Food Can Trigger an Asthma Attack: Up to 10% of Cases,", Family Practice News, (1997); 60.

54 Rietz, Dave, viewed 12 January, 2009, http://www.rense.com/general26/milk.htm

55 Rietz, Dave, viewed 12 January, 2009, http://www.rense.com/general26/milk.htm

56 American Heart Association, viewed 12 January, 2009, http://www.americanheart.org/Heart_and_Stroke_A_Z_Guide/vegdiet.html

57 Cohen, Robert, viewed 12 January, 2009, http://www.notmilk.com

58 Amy Joy Lanou, PhD, Susan E Berkow, PhD CN and Neal D. Barnard, MD. "Calcium, Dairy Products and Bone Health in Children and Young Adults: A reevaluation." Pediatrics 115.3 (2005) pages 736-743

59 Amy Joy Lanou, PhD, Susan E Berkow, PhD CN and Neal D. Barnard, MD. "Calcium, Dairy Products and Bone Health in Children and Young Adults: A reevaluation." Pediatrics 115.3 (2005) pages 736-743

60 Viewed 11 January, 2009, www.rense.com/general26/milk.htm

61 Marteau, et al, (1996) "Effects of Lactobacillus acidophilus strain LA1 on serum concentration and jejunal secretions of immunoglobulins and serum proteins in healthy humans." In SOMED 21st Intl. Congress on microbial ecology and disease, Paris, October 28-30, 1996.

62 Hayden, David, http://davidhayden.com/blog/dave/archive/2005/06/13/1418.aspx

63 Diagnose Me.com, 3 November, 2008, viewed 11 December, 2009, http://www.diagnose-me.com/treat/T136795.html

64 Pearce, Matthew, viewed 23 January, 2009, http://twgr.blogspot.com/2006/01/is-coffee-poison.html

65 Penis Health.com, "Home Remedies for Erectile Dysfunction", viewed 1 January, 2009, www.penishealth.com/article/home-remedies-for-erectile-dysfunction.html

66 Matthias B. Schulze, DrPH; JoAnn E. Manson, MD; David S. Ludwig, MD; Graham A. Colditz, MD; Meir J. Stampfer, MD; Walter C. Willett, MD; Frank B. Hu, MD, "Sugar-Sweetened Beverages, Weight Gain, and Incidence of Type 2 Diabetes in Young and Middle-Aged Women", 25 August 2004, viewed 12 January, 2009, http://jama.ama-assn.org/cgi/content/abstract/292/8/927,

67 Globe and Mail, "Controversial chemical found in at least 84% of canned pop sold in Canada", 4 March, 2009

68 Kimmon, Dama, "New link between soft drinks and weight gain", University of Cincinnati, 31 July, 2005, Viewed 12 January, 2009, http://www.medicalnewstoday.com/articles/28346.php

69 Pick, Marcelle, OB/GYN NP, "Diet Soda-How Healthy is it?" 20 June, 2006, Viewed 11 December, 2009, http://www.womentowomen.com/nutritionandweightloss/dietsoda.aspx

70 Oklahoma Fit Kids Association, www.fitkidsok.org, Viewed 11 January, 2009, www.fitkidsok.org

71 Group, Dr. Edward, "The Health Dangers of Energy Drinks", Global Healing Center Blog, June 14, 2008, viewed 12 January, 2009, http://www.ghchealth.com/natural-health/the-health-dangers-of-energy-drinks

72 "Progress Against Cancer at Risk", American Cancer Society, 10 April, 2007, viewed 11 January, 2009, http://www.cancer.org/docroot/NWS/content/NWS_1_1x_ACS_Report_Progress_Against_Cancer_at_Risk.asp

73 "How Alcohol Affects Vital Organs", 18 September, 2008, Viewed 12 January, 2009 http://www.searchtempoblog.com/index.php/page/2/

74 "Mediterranean diet: Choose this heart-healthy diet option", Viewed 16 January, 2009 http://www.mayoclinic.com/health/mediterranean-diet/CL00011

75 Adams, Mike, "Nurses Recommend Aluminum-Free Deodorants", 26 July, 2005, Viewed 30 January, 2009, http://www.naturalnews.com/009969.html